MRCPsych Pa

600 MCQs and EMIs

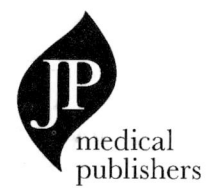

JP medical publishers

MRCPsych Paper B

600 MCQs and EMIs

Ashok G Patel MBBS DPM FRCPsych
Consultant in General Adult Psychiatry (retired)
South Essex Partnership University NHS Foundation Trust
Luton, UK

Roshelle Ramkisson MBBS MRCPsych MSc (Health and Public Leadership)
PGDip Psychiatry MDCH
Consultant in Child and Adolescent Psychiatry
Pennine Care NHS Foundation Trust
Royal Oldham Hospital
Oldham, UK

Madhavan Seshadri MBBS DPM MRCPsych PG Cert ME
Consultant in General Adult Psychiatry
Recovery Team North
2gether NHS Foundation Trust
Leominster, UK

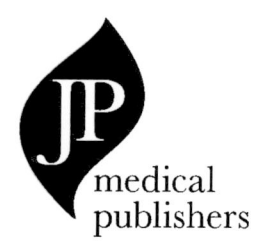

JP medical publishers

London • Philadelphia • Panama City • New Delhi

© 2015 JP Medical Ltd.
Published by JP Medical Ltd
83 Victoria Street, London SW1H 0HW, UK
Tel: +44 (0)20 3170 8910   Fax: +44 (0)20 3008 6180
Email: info@jpmedpub.com   Web: www.jpmedpub.com

The rights of Ashok G Patel, Roshelle Ramkisson and Madhavan Seshadri to be identified as editors of this work have been asserted by them in accordance with the Copyright, Designs and Patents Act 1988.

All rights reserved. No part of this publication may be reproduced, stored or transmitted in any form or by any means, electronic, mechanical, photocopying, recording or otherwise, except as permitted by the UK Copyright, Designs and Patents Act 1988, without the prior permission in writing of the publishers. Permissions may be sought directly from JP Medical Ltd at the address printed above.

All brand names and product names used in this book are trade names, service marks, trademarks or registered trademarks of their respective owners. The publisher is not associated with any product or vendor mentioned in this book.

Medical knowledge and practice change constantly. This book is designed to provide accurate, authoritative information about the subject matter in question. However, readers are advised to check the most current information available on procedures included and check information from the manufacturer of each product to be administered, to verify the recommended dose, formula, method and duration of administration, adverse effects and contraindications. It is the responsibility of the practitioner to take all appropriate safety precautions. Neither the publisher nor the editors assume any liability for any injury and/or damage to persons or property arising from or related to use of material in this book.

This book is sold on the understanding that the publisher is not engaged in providing professional medical services. If such advice or services are required, the services of a competent medical professional should be sought.

Every effort has been made where necessary to contact holders of copyright to obtain permission to reproduce copyright material. If any have been inadvertently overlooked, the publisher will be pleased to make the necessary arrangements at the first opportunity.

ISBN: 978-1-909836-20-4

British Library Cataloguing in Publication Data
A catalogue record for this book is available from the British Library

Library of Congress Cataloging in Publication Data
A catalog record for this book is available from the Library of Congress

Commissioning Editor:	Steffan Clements
Editorial Assistant:	Katie Pattullo
Design:	Designers Collective Ltd

Typeset, printed and bound in India.

Preface

The MRCPsych examinations are extremely challenging, and candidates must be meticulous in their preparation if they are to stand any chance of success. Understanding this principle has been fundamental during our preparation of this book, and we have endeavoured to provide sufficient revision material for each element of the curriculum. We are confident that by using this book, readers will be well armed to face the new Paper B exam.

In order to facilitate revision, we have mapped the questions in the first two chapters to the MRCPsych curriculum. The third chapter is intentionally unstructured, and has been included to provide a mock exam representative of Paper B, which readers can use to practise under exam conditions. All questions are based on the curriculum and thorough answers have been provided to explain the rationale behind each correct answer option.

The burden of editorship has been wisely spread to harness varied expertise. In psychiatry, innovation in practice tends to be evolutionary rather than revolutionary, and much of our knowledge remains to be translated into practical innovations in patient care. It is our intention that this book will help psychiatry trainees not only to pass the MRCPsych Paper B examination, but also to improve their patient care. We believe that the book will assist trainees, trainers, educational and clinical supervisors, College tutors, Directors of Medical Education, SAS tutors and Training Programme Directors in preparation for the MRCPsych examinations.

Ashok G Patel
Roshelle Ramkisson
Madhavan Seshadri
December 2014

Contents

Preface		v
Contributors		ix
Chapter 1	**Mock Exam: 1**	**1**
	Questions: MCQs	1
	Questions: EMIs	24
	Answers: MCQs	32
	Answers: EMIs	60
Chapter 2	**Mock Exam: 2**	**73**
	Questions: MCQs	73
	Questions: EMIs	97
	Answers: MCQs	106
	Answers: EMIs	133
Chapter 3	**Mock Exam: 3**	**145**
	Questions: MCQs	145
	Questions: EMIs	166
	Answers: MCQs	174
	Answers: EMIs	202

Contributors

Dr Samir Shah MBBS MRCPsych MSc MDCH
Consultant in General Adult Psychiatry
Cheshire and Wirral Partnership NHS Foundation Trust
Jocelyn Solly Resource Centre
Macclesfield, UK

Dinesh Khanna MBBS MSc MRCPsych
Consultant in Child and Adolescent Psychiatry
Cumbria Partnership NHS Foundation Trust
Kinta House Annex
Kendal, UK

Gursharan Lal Kashyap MBBS DCH MD MRCPsych
Specialty Registrar in Psychiatry
South Essex Partnership University NHS Foundation Trust
Bedford Hospital
Bedford, UK

Hany El-Mataal MBChB MRCPsych
Consultant in Forensic Psychiatry
Greater Manchester West NHS Foundation Trust
Prestwich Hospital
Manchester, UK

Komal A Patel BSc MBChB MRCS
Core Trainee in Surgery
Medway Maritime Hospital
Gillingham, UK

Krishna Madhusudhan MBBS MRCPsych
Consultant in Child and Adolescent Psychiatry
Black Country NHS Partnership Foundation Trust
Child and Adolescent Mental Health Service (CAMHS)
West Bromwich, UK

Louise Draper BSc MBChB MRCPsych PGDip
Consultant in Child and Adolescent Psychiatry
Alder Hey Children's NHS Foundation Trust
Alder Hey Children's Hospital
Liverpool, UK

Syed Ashraf MBBS PGCHM
Specialty Doctor in Psychiatry
South Essex Partnership University NHS Foundation Trust
Bedford Hospital
Bedford, UK

Sanjith Kamath MBBS MRCPsych
Consultant in General Adult Psychiatry
St Andrews Healthcare
Northampton, UK

Chapter 1

Mock Exam: 1

Questions: MCQs

For each question, select one answer option

ORGANISATION AND DELIVERY OF PSYCHIATRIC SERVICES

1. Which one of the following staff and training statements is a standard requirement for ECT treatment, according to the Electroconvulsive Therapy Accreditation Service (ECTAS)?

   A   There should be at least two trained nurses in the treatment area
   B   There should be at least one trained nurse in the recovery area
   C   There can be a different ECT team in clinic every week
   D   The lead ECT nurse develops protocols for ECT prescription
   E   One competent person should be present in cardiopulmonary resuscitation for every two unconscious patients

2. Which one of the following statements about the provision of information on ECT to patients is correct, according to the Electroconvulsive Therapy Accreditation Service (ECTAS)?

   A   Consent can be obtained by the ECT lead nurse
   B   An 'ECT rights about consent to treatment' leaflet is provided to detained patients
   C   ECT information should be provided verbally
   D   An explanation on why ECT does not affect cognition should be provided
   E   There is no need to document capacity assessment for informal patients

3. Which one of the following clinical predictors is a response to phototherapy?

   A   Diurnal variation in mood
   B   Increased appetite
   C   Morning slump in energy
   D   Reduced sleep
   E   Winter weight loss

4. You are treating a 34-year-old female patient who suffers from recurrent depressive disorder. She is not responding to conventional medication. She does not want ECT. She came to your clinic today enquiring about rTMS (transcranial magnetic stimulation). Which one of the following statements about rTMS is true?

   A   A small dose of electric current is passed through the brain in rTMS
   B   Patient needs to be anaesthetised during rTMS.
   C   rTMS stands for rhythmic transcranial magnetic stimulation.
   D   The effectiveness of rTMS is measured by the duration of seizures.
   E   The intensity of rTMS is usually set as a percentage of the patient's motor threshold

Mock Exam: 1

5. Which one of the following conditions is a clinical indication for psychosurgery?

    A Bipolar affective disorder
    B Bulimia nervosa
    C Obsessive compulsive disorder
    D Post-traumatic stress disorder
    E Schizophrenia

6. Which of the following is considered the best established approach to assess psychiatric needs?

    A Eysenck Personality Questionnaire
    B General health questionnaire
    C Milton Clinical Multi-axial Inventory
    D Recovery Star
    E The Camberwell Assessment of Need

7. According to guidance on the Mental Capacity Act (2005) from the Crown Prosecution Service there are three categories of offences against people with a mental disorder. Which one of the following statements is correct?

    A An offence against someone with a mental disorder who is unable to refuse
    B An offence against someone in whom there is a suspicion of mental disorder
    C It is not an offence if sexual activity is with consent in someone with serious mental disorder
    D Offence against someone with a mental disorder who is unable to refuse
    E In all these offences, legal definition of mental disorder is different to that in the Mental Health Act 1983 (amended 2007)

8. You are a ST4 Trainee working in drug and alcohol services. The neurologist from the county hospital has referred a 42-year-old man diagnosed with an alcohol-related seizure. You assess him in the clinic. He has no features of alcohol or substance dependence. This is an isolated event and he has never suffered from epilepsy. The patient wants to know whether he can drive his car to work. Which one of the following would you recommned?

    A Referral to epilepsy guidance related to driving
    B The patient may continue driving and need not inform the DVLA as this is an isolated alcohol-related seizure.
    C The patient may continue driving but should inform the DVLA as this is an isolated alcohol-related seizure.
    D The patient should stop driving for at least 6 months and inform the DVLA as this is an isolated alcohol-related seizure.
    E Patient should stop driving for at least 3 months and inform the DVLA as this is an isolated alcohol-related seizure.

9. Which one of the following is the only ever mental health-related incident referred to as a 'never event' in England?

    A Death of a patient at the time of receiving ECT.
    B Death of a patient treated with high-dose antipsychotics.
    C Inpatient suicide by hanging using a non-collapsible curtain rail.
    D Serial killing by a patient with schizophrenia.
    E Suicide by hanging using a non-collapsible curtain rail.

RESEARCH METHODS, STATISTICS, CRITICAL REVIEW AND EVIDENCE-BASED PRACTICE

Answer questions 10–14 using the following information

A study was carried out to compare an antidepressant A with a control drug B. There were around 200 patients in each group; 190 patients improved on drug A whereas 120 patients improved with drug B (**Table 1.1**).

Table 1.1 Drug comparison study

Drug	Improved (remission)	Not improved
A (antidepressant)	190	10
B (control)	120	80

10. What is the remission rate of depression for drug A?

    A 0.2
    B 0.4
    C 0.6
    D 0.95
    E 1

11. What is the remission rate of depression for drug B?

    A 0.3
    B 0.5
    C 0.6
    D 0.9
    E 1.2

12. What is the absolute benefit increase?

    A 0.15
    B 0.25
    C 0.35
    D 0.45
    E 0.55

13. What is the number needed to treat (NNT) for drug A?

    A 1
    B 3
    C 5
    D 10
    E 20

14. What term is used when the null hypothesis is rejected even though it is true?

    A   Power
    B   Probability
    C   Standard deviation
    D   Type 1 error
    E   Type 2 error

For each question, select one answer option

15. What term is used when the null hypothesis is accepted even though it is false?

    A   Accuracy
    B   False positive
    C   Standard error
    D   Type 1 error
    E   Type 2 error

16. What is the average distance from the mean in a normal distribution?

    A   Negative skewed
    B   Positive skewed
    C   Standard deviation (SD)
    D   Standard error
    E   Variable

17. What is an approximate population score within three standard deviations of a normal distribution?

    A   95.7%
    B   96.7%
    C   97.7%
    D   98.8%
    E   99.7%

18. What is the ability to detect differences between groups if they are truly present known as?

    A   α
    B   β
    C   Effect size
    D   Power
    E   Probability

19. Which of the following non-parametric tests is used to compare two unpaired groups independently?

    A   Mann–Whitney U test
    B   McNemar's test
    C   Student's t-test
    D   Wilcoxon's rank sum test
    E χ^2 test

20. Which of the following parametric statistical tests is used in comparing more than two groups?

    A   Analysis of variance (ANOVA)
    B   Kruskal–Wallis analysis of variance
    C   Paired Student's t-test
    D   Wilcoxon's rank sum test
    E χ^2 test

Questions: MCQs

21. Which of the following p values (probability) would be considered statistically significant?

    A ≥0.04
    B ≥0.06
    C ≥0.08
    D ≥0.10
    E ≥0.50

22. What is the range for a linear correlation?

    A −0.01 to + 0.01
    B −0.05 to + 0.05
    C −0.1 to + 0.1
    D −1 to + 1
    E −1.5 to + 1.5

23. If the mean = 4, standard deviation 1.4 and n =16, what is the 95% confidence interval?

    A 4 ± 0.15
    B 4 ± 0.68
    C 4 ± 2.21
    D 4 ± 2.31
    E 4 ± 5.6

24. What is subjective assessment when the item appears to measure the desired qualities?

    A Face validity
    B Concurrent validity
    C Construct validity
    D Convergent validity
    E Divergent validity

25. What type of validity assesses the extent to which a depression questionnaire actually measures depression?

    A Content validity
    B Construct validity
    C Convergent validity
    D Discriminant validity
    E Predictive validity

26. Which of the following assesses the consistency of items within a scale or subscale?

    A Interobserver reliability
    B Internal consistency
    C Intraclass correlation coefficient
    D Intraobserver reliability (test–re-test)
    E κ

27. Which bias occurs in a hospital-based study about the relationship between exposure and disease?

    A Berkson's bias
    B Diagnostic purity bias
    C Historical control bias
    D Membership bias
    E Referral filter bias

28. What type of reliability is measured by an intraclass correlation?

    A   Construct reliability
    B   Internal consistency reliability
    C   Interobserver reliability
    D   Split-half reliability
    E   Test-re-test reliability

29. What is the name given to a situation in which the observation is influenced by observer knowledge?

    A   Demand effect
    B   Domino effect
    C   Halo effect
    D   Hawthorne's effect
    E   Placebo effect

30. What is Neyman's bias also known as?

    A   Berkson's bias
    B   Confounding bias
    C   Information bias
    D   Prevalence–incidence bias
    E   Publication bias

31. Which of the following is a critically appraised database?

    A   Clinical Practice Guidelines
    B   Cochrane Library
    C   EMBASE
    D   PsycINFO
    E   PubMed

32. According to current evidence, in which of the following disorders do omega-3 essential fatty acids have a role in treatment?

    A   Affective disorders
    B   Alcohol misuse
    C   Anxiety disorders
    D   Psychotic disorders
    E   Personality disorders

33. A clinical drug study was conducted to evaluate the efficacy of aripiprazole in patients with recurrent depersonalisation–derealisation. It was necessary to calculate the number of participants needed in the study to demonstrate a meaningful effect and the α (x) level was set at 0.01. Which of the following is correct?

    A   Ten per cent of the participants in the study will show an absence of clinical effect.
    B   If $x = 0.01$, there is a probability of 1% that the null hypothesis is wrongly rejected.
    C   It is the maximum threshold for defining clinical efficacy and therefore the clinical significance in the study.
    D   It is the minimum threshold for defining clinical efficacy and therefore the clinical significance in the study.
    E   There is a probability of a type 2 error.

34. In an audit of the length of stay in a hospital, the outcome was presented as median days. However, the analysed data showed many observations that were substantially higher than the median. Which of the following is correct?

   A   Mean > median
   B   Mean = median
   C   Mode = median
   D   Mode = mean
   E   Mode ≥ median

35. In conducting randomised controlled trials (RCTs), it is necessary to observe certain requirements to obtain meaningful results. The randomisation sequence is protected throughout the study until the last participant has been enrolled in the study. What is this known as?

   A   Allocation concealment
   B   Blinding
   C   Masking
   D   Matching
   E   Publication bias

36. In a meta-analysis, the results of different studies are combined to detect treatment effects. However, this could be confounded by heterogeneity in the studies. Which of the following methods is used to assess heterogeneity?

   A   Minimisation
   B   Paired Student's t-statistics
   C   Q statistics
   D   Randomisation
   E   Stratification

37. A multicentre randomised controlled trial of a new compound thought to be an antidepressant was planned. This trial had strict inclusion criteria of hospitalised patients. Which of the following properties of this trial is most likely to be affected by strict inclusion criteria?

   A   Accuracy of the results
   B   Clinical significance of the results
   C   Desirability of the results
   D   Precision of the results
   E   Statistical significance of the results

38. A psychiatric trainee was interested in studying whether pregnant mothers who took amphetamines increased the risk of attention deficit hyperactivity disorder (ADHD) in their offspring. Which of the following statements represents the null hypothesis?

   A   Taking amphetamines during pregnancy does not increase the risk of ADHD in the child.
   B   Taking amphetamines during pregnancy increases the risk of ADHD in the child.
   C   Taking amphetamines during pregnancy decreases the risk of ADHD in the child.
   D   Taking amphetamines during pregnancy has no bearing on the risk of ADHD in the child.
   E   Taking amphetamines during pregnancy increases the risk of ADHD in the mother.

39. Which of the following is the most important methodological challenge when conducting a cohort study?

   A   Concealment of the allocation
   B   Identifying a suitable control group
   C   Identifying a suitable study group
   D   Publication bias
   E   Statistical analysis of the findings

Answer questions 40–42 by using the following information

A 4-week RCT of aripiprazole in patients with schizophrenia was conducted; 150 patients were recruited in the aripiprazole group and 150 patients in the placebo group. Of these, 125 patients in each group completed the study. Using categorical measures of treatment response, it was reported that 70% of patients in the aripiprazole group improved whereas only 20% in the placebo group improved.

40. What is the relative risk reduction from using aripiprazole?

    A   1.5
    B   2.5
    C   3.5
    D   4.5
    E   5.5

41. Using the results from the above study, what is the number needed to treat (NNT) for patients receiving aripiprazole compared with placebo?

    A   2
    B   3
    C   4
    D   5
    E   6

42. What is the odds ratio of having a response using a per protocol analysis of primary outcome in the above study?

    A   8
    B   9.3
    C   11.5
    D   12.5
    E   13.5

For each question, select one answer option

43. Which of the following statements is a limitation of the cross-sectional studies?

    A   Cross-sectional studies are prone to recollection bias.
    B   Cross-sectional studies require fewer patients.
    C   Finding a control group is very difficult.
    C   These studies are prohibitively expensive.
    D   The direction of the effect cannot be determined.

44. In the hierarchy of levels of evidence-based medicine, which of these statements is correct?

    A   An individual case–control study is on a higher level than an outcome research study.
    B   Review of case–control studies is higher than of individual cohort studies.
    C   Systematic reviews of RCTs are above systematic reviews of cohort studies.
    D   Systematic reviews of cohort studies are lower than outcome research studies
    E   Systematic reviews of cohort studies are higher than individual RCTs.

45. In the treatment of eating disorders in adolescents, family interventions were given a grade B recommendation of evidence. What type of studies does this refer to?

    A   Individual RCTs
    B   Individual case–control studies
    C   Systematic review of cohort studies

D Systematic review of case–control studies
E Systematic review of RCTs

46. Which of the following phenomena is described by Hawthorne's effect?

    A Individuals show improvement because they are aware of their participation in research.
    B Smaller sample size gives false-positive results.
    C There is a tendency for the result to be positive just by chance.
    D The effect sizes decrease as studies are replicated.
    E Unknown confounders modify the results.

47. Which of the following statements represents an advantage of an intention-to-treat analysis?

    A It stops the selection biases from creeping back into the study.
    B It allows better analysis of the data.
    C It can make up numbers if there are a large number of dropouts.
    D It gives more accurate results.
    E It is ethical to include the dropouts in the final analysis.

48. Which of the following statements about replication studies is correct?

    A Replication studies are easily published.
    B Replication studies get ethical approval easily.
    C Replication studies must be done using exactly the same methods as in the original study.
    D Replication studies on a different population help to add weight to the findings.
    E Undertaking a replication study is better than doing an original study.

49. Which of the following statements about publication bias is correct?

    A Publishers show bias towards what interests their publications.
    B Research with better methodology has a higher chance of being published.
    C Research with positive results has a higher chance of being published
    D Research with well-known experts has a higher chance of being published
    E Researchers use contacts to get their findings published.

50. Which of the following statements about a binary variable is correct?

    A A variable can take any value within a limited range.
    B A variable describes a group of people.
    C Another variable cannot be converted to binary variable.
    D It is also known as a dichotomous variable.
    E It is also known as an ordinal variable.

51. Which of the following statements about the Paediatric OCD Treatment Study (POTS) is correct?

    A It was conducted in three academic centres between 1997 and 2002.
    B It was conducted for a period of 8 weeks.
    C It was conducted in Canada.
    D It was conducted to compare CBT with fluoxetine in treatment of OCD.
    E The findings suggested that fluoxetine was better than CBT.

52. Which of the following statements about the findings in the CAFÉ (Comparison of Atypicals in First Episode of psychosis) trial is correct?

    A All-cause discontinuation was the primary outcome measure.
    B Compared with other antipsychotics, quetiapine was more potent than others in treating the illness.
    C A greater reduction in overall PANSS scores was seen in participants treated with quetiapine.
    D Of the three antipsychotics compared, quetiapine was associated with the smallest elevations in fasting triglyceride and cholesterol levels
    E Safety and tolerability were also a primary measure.

53. What does CUtLASS 1 stand for?

    A Cost of Universally used Latest Antipsychotics in Schizophrenia Study 1
    B Cost Utility of the Latest Antipsychotics in Schizophrenia Study 1
    C Creating Universally used Latest Antipsychotics in Schizophrenia Study 1
    D Cutting the Universal use of Latest Antipsychotics in Schizophrenia Study 1
    E Cutting Universally used Latest Antipsychotics in Schizophrenia Study 1

54. Which of the following statements about CUtLASS 1 is correct?

    A Clozapine and olanzapine were two of the second-generation antipsychotics.
    B Depot preparations were excluded from the study design.
    C More than 300 participants were assessed during the study.
    D One of the outcome measures included scores of quality-of-life scales.
    E Participants were from hospitals in the NHS and private sector in England

55. The objective of the research is to explore, interpret or obtain a deeper understanding of a particular clinical issue. Which of the following methods is it most appropriate to use?

    A Case–control study
    B Prospective cohort study
    C Qualitative research
    D Quantitative research
    E Randomised controlled trial

56. Which of the following is used to compare treatments when the effect of interventions can be expressed in terms of one main variable?

    A Cost-benefit analysis
    B Cost-effectiveness analysis
    C Cost-hybridisation analysis
    D Cost-minimisation analysis
    E Cost–utility analysis

57. Which of the following is the extent to which the results of a study are generalisable or applicable to a particular target population?

    A Accuracy
    B External validity
    C Internal validity
    D Methodological quality
    E Precision

GENERAL ADULT PSYCHIATRY

58. Which of the following conditions can reliably be assessed by the Bush–Francis scale?

    A Acute psychosis
    B Catatonia
    C Delirium
    D Extrapyramidal side effects
    E Opioid withdrawal symptoms

59. A 32-year-old man presented with a 3-month history of depressed mood, loss of energy, anhedonia, and disturbed appetite and sleep. He was also not able to concentrate. For the last 2 months, he had been experiencing auditory hallucinations asking him to take his own life. He

thought that people looked at him when he went out and had become increasingly withdrawn. What is the single most likely diagnosis?

- A Bipolar affective disorder, current episode severe depression with psychotic symptoms
- B Depressive disorder with psychotic symptoms
- C Post-schizophrenic depression
- D Schizoaffective disorder
- E Schizophrenia

60. In which of the following is Ganser's syndrome more likely to be seen?

- A Bipolar affective disorder
- B Dementia
- C Factitious disorder
- D Prisoners awaiting trial
- E Schizophrenia

61. A 21-year-old woman was known to have anorexia nervosa. Which of the following metabolic disturbances is the most likely to be found in this patient?

- A Hyperkalaemia
- B Impaired glucose tolerance
- C Increased luteinising hormone (LH) levels
- D Increased somatomedin C
- E Reduced cortisol levels

62. A 22-year-old man with schizophrenia was admitted to an assessment ward. He was reported to be making good progress. However, his behaviour worsened whenever he returned from home leave. In the ward round, his mother complained that he was very lazy. What is the most appropriate next step to help this patient?

- A Cognitive–behavioural therapy (CBT)
- B Community treatment order under the Mental Health Act
- C Counselling
- D Family therapy
- E Interpersonal therapy

63. Which of the following subtypes of schizophrenia is classified in DSM-IV but not ICD-10?

- A Disorganised schizophrenia
- B Hebephrenic schizophrenia
- C Post-schizophrenic depression
- D Residual schizophrenia
- E Undifferentiated schizophrenia

64. Over the past 3 years, a 20-year-old man was becoming increasingly isolated. He spent most of his time in his room and there was some evidence of self-neglect. This was associated with a marked decline in his educational performance and inability to hold any job due to difficulty in planning and making decisions. What is the most likely diagnosis?

- A Asperger's syndrome
- B Autism
- C Catatonic personality disorder
- D Schizoid personality disorder
- E Simple schizophrenia

65. Which of the following is considered Valliant's predictor of good prognosis in schizophrenia?

- A Absence of stressful precipitating factor
- B Absence of affective symptoms

    C   Chronic onset
    D   Family history of depression
    E   Schizoid traits

66. A 57-year-old man was found wandering the streets by police. He was brought to the accident and emergency department (A&E). He was considered to be in a fugue state. Which of the following is the correct statement about fugue states?

    A   Depressed mood is an extremely rare antecedent for a psychogenic fugue state.
    B   A fugue state is a syndrome consisting of a gradual loss of all autobiographical memories and knowledge of personal identity.
    C   A fugue state is usually associated with a period of wandering, for which there is a subsequent amnesic gap on recovery.
    D   Fugue states are usually not preceded by a severe precipitating stress.
    E   Fugue states are similar to transient global amnesia or transient epileptic amnesia in that the person does not know whom he or she is.

67. A 45-year-old man with a long history of alcohol dependence was diagnosed with Wernicke–Korsakoff syndrome. Which of the following statements about his condition is correct?

    A   False memories are jumbled up and retrieved appropriately, within a temporal context.
    B   It is found more commonly *post mortem* in people with alcohol problems than it is diagnosed in life.
    C   It is the result of nutritional depletion, namely a vitamin C deficiency.
    D   The disorder almost always has an acute onset.
    E   There is usually an anterograde memory loss.

68. A 27-year-old woman was brought to A&E. She was considered to have herpes encephalitis. Which of the following statements about herpes encephalitis is correct?

    A   Herpes encephalitis can give rise to a severe form of amnesic syndrome.
    B   Neuropathological and neuroimaging studies show that there is an extensive bilateral occipital lobe damage.
    C   Seizures are a common occurrence.
    D   The fully developed clinical picture with neck rigidity, vomiting, and motor and sensory deficits almost always occurs during the first week.
    E   The minority of cases are said to be primary infections.

69. A 34-year-old woman was considered to have intermittent uncontrollable, pathological laughter and crying spells. She was otherwise reported to be symptom free. Which of the following statements about this condition is correct?

    A   Absence of voluntary control on facial expressions
    B   Associated mood changes exaggerate response
    C   Duloxetine is an effective treatment
    D   Presence of incongruent affect
    E   Requires specific stimuli to precipitate the condition

70. A 48-year-old woman had had multiple sclerosis for some years now. She enquired about the neuropsychiatric aspects of her condition of which she should be aware. Which of the following is a neuropsychiatric manifestation of multiple sclerosis?

    A   The patient can present with subcortical dementia.
    B   Hypomania due to steroids is more likely in patients with a family history of an affective disorder.
    C   The late onset of illness is associated with a high risk of suicide.

D   The lifetime prevalence of depression is 14%.
E   Psychosis is three times more common than in the general population.

71. A 34-year-old woman presented with tiredness for more than a year. She had been off sick for more than 6 months and was unable to carry on with her routine activities. She had poor concentration, poor memory, headaches, sore throat and joint pains. What is the most likely diagnosis?

    A   Chronic fatigue syndrome
    B   Depression
    C   Hypothyroidism
    D   Factitious disorder
    E   Somatisation disorder

72. Schizotaxia is:

    A   Ataxia in schizophrenia
    B   Familial schizotypal disorder
    C   Genetic constitution increasing vulnerability to schizophrenia
    D   Neuropsychiatric manifestations in schizophrenia
    E   Slow cognitive decline in schizophrenia

73. Which of the following is a correct match of medical condition associated with a secondary sleep problem?

    A   Dementia–nocturnal myoclonus
    B   Epilepsy–parasomnias
    C   Huntington's disease–hypersomnia
    D   Kleine–Levin syndrome–difficulty initiating sleep
    E   Parkinsonism–sun downing

74. In which of the following is the 'match box' or 'pill bottle' sign seen?

    A   Delusions involving the skin
    B   Delusions of body odour
    C   Delusions of sexually transmitted infection
    D   Delusions of ugliness
    E   Pyromania

75. A 37-year-old man with a persistent delusional disorder attended your outpatient clinic. You discussed his treatment options and prognosis with him. Which of the following is a correct statement about this?

    A   A delusional system ameliorates after just 2–3 months.
    B   The maintenance antipsychotic dose is usually very high.
    C   Once treated successfully, if the patient stops medication he is likely to remain stable for around 6–12 months before he may relapse.
    D   Overall, the best-attested treatment result refers to somatic subtype.
    E   Recovery is often very slow.

76. In which of the following conditions is an accentuation of a normal EEG seen?

    A   Alzheimer's disease
    B   Creutzfeldt–Jakob disease
    C   Huntington's disease
    D   Presenile Alzheimer's disease
    E   Pseudo-dementia

Mock Exam: 1

77. A 40-year-old man was recently diagnosed with Wilson's disease. He enquired about the possible psychiatric manifestations of his condition of which he should be aware. Which of the following is correct about Wilson's disease?

    A Cognitive impairment
    B Depression
    C Disorientation
    D Personality change and incongruous behaviour
    E Psychotic behaviour

78. A 62-year-old woman with systemic lupus erythematosus (SLE) was referred to your outpatient clinic. She enquired about the possible neuropsychiatric manifestations of her condition. Which of the following statements about SLE is correct?

    A Headaches are most uncommon.
    B They are characteristic features of SLE.
    C They are usually long-term manifestations.
    D They show a tendency to appear in the later stages of the disease.
    E They usually reoccur when there are no other systemic features.

79. A 42-year-old woman with hypothyroidism presented in your outpatient clinic. She would like to know about the neuropsychiatric manifestations of her condition. Which of the following statements about hypothyroidism is correct?

    A Auditory hallucinations are less common than other types of perceptual abnormalities.
    B Depression with psychotic symptoms responds readily to treatment with psychotropic medications.
    C Memory is intact to a large extent in the early stages.
    D Mood is depressed rather than manic.
    E Paranoid features figure prominently in psychosis.

80. A 52-year-old woman with Cushing's syndrome presented in your outpatient clinic. She would like to discuss the psychiatric manifestations of her condition. Which of the following statements about Cushing's syndrome is correct?

    A Depression is the most common psychiatric presentation in Cushing's syndrome due to pituitary involvement.
    B Depression is the most common psychiatric presentation in Cushing's syndrome due to adrenal carcinoma or adenoma.
    C Psychiatric disturbances are found in only 20–25% of cases.
    D Psychosis often presents without any flavour of paranoia but mainly with auditory hallucinations.
    E Psychotic depression is the most common manifestation.

81. A 39-year-old man presented in the initial stage of Huntington's disease in your outpatient clinic. He wanted to know about the psychiatric manifestations and likely prognosis of his condition. Which of the following statements is correct?

    A Dementia precedes involuntary movements.
    B It follows a more severe course when the onset is early.
    C Psychiatric changes usually occur once the diagnosis has been fully established.
    D The ratio of incidence is male:female = 6:1.
    E The abnormal movements continue to a lesser extent during sleep.

82. Which of the following statements about parasuicide is correct?

    A It is usually an impulsive act.
    B Life events are common in the 6 months before an act of parasuicide.

C   Most cases of parasuicide are associated with malingering.
D   Parasuicide was first defined by Melanie Klein.
E   A person injures him- or herself by taking a substance in a quantity that is less than the therapeutic dose.

83. A 29-year-old woman with body dysmorphic disorder (BDD) attended your clinic for a review. She would like to learn more about her condition. Which of the following statements about BDD is correct?

   A   Anorexia nervosa does not fulfil the diagnostic criteria for BDD.
   B   In psychodynamic terms, BDD has not been considered to represent an unconscious displacement on to body parts of sexual or emotional conflicts, or of general feelings of inferiority, poor self-image or guilt.
   C   It is a delusional belief of slight or perceived defect of one's body.
   D   Studies of college students have suggested that a quarter meet DSM-IV criteria for BDD.
   E   The most common age of onset is the third decade of life.

84. A 35-year-old woman attended your clinic with multiple psychosomatic symptoms. Which of the following statements is least likely to describe the medically unexplained physical symptoms?

   A   About a quarter of new consultations in secondary care will be for medically unexplained symptoms.
   B   In any week, 60–80% of healthy people experience bodily symptoms.
   C   Most patients in clinical practice with unexplained physical symptoms have either an undifferentiated somatoform disorder or a primary psychiatric disorder.
   D   Somatic symptoms of pain in the face are considered psychodynamically equivalent to an emotional 'slap in the face'.
   E   Symptoms are transient but a third persist and cause distress and disability.

85. A 21-year-old man was diagnosed with schizophrenia. He was worried about his twin brother becoming mentally ill. What is the likely risk of developing schizophrenia in the identical twin of a person with schizophrenia?

   A   0–10%
   B   10–20%
   C   20–30%
   D   30–40%
   E   40–65%

86. A 24-year-old woman was diagnosed with pseudo-seizures. Which of the following statements about this condition is correct?

   A   Of patients 40–50% have coexisting epilepsy.
   B   Clinical observation can differentiate easily between pseudo-seizures and seizures.
   C   They are a post-ictal impaired papillary reflex.
   D   They are a post-ictal decrease in prolactin concentration.
   E   Urinary incontinence can occur in this condition.

87. Which of the following is a characteristic feature of the Gastaut–Geschwind syndrome?

   A   Hyperreligiosity
   B   Hypersexuality
   C   Hypographia
   D   Mainly seen in absent seizure
   E   Tangential

OLD AGE PSYCHIATRY

88. A 76-year-old woman presented in your outpatient clinic with paranoid symptoms and general decline in her personal hygiene. A diagnosis of late-onset schizophrenia was considered as most likely in the absence of any organic brain pathology. Which of the following is correct?

   A Better response to antipsychotics
   B Increased likelihood of affective blunting
   C Increased likelihood of formal thought disorder
   D Less risk of developing tardive dyskinesia
   E More negative than positive symptoms

89. A 68-year-old man had had a mental disorder for a long time. He wished to discuss the long-term implications of his condition because he had read that he carried an increased risk for vascular disease in later life. Which of the following disorders is he most likely to have at present?

   A Bipolar affective disorder
   B Generalised anxiety disorder
   C Obsessive–compulsive disorder
   D Recurrent depression
   E Schizophrenia

90. A 70-year-old woman had treatment-resistant depression. She consented to a course of electroconvulsive therapy (ECT). Which of the following factors leads to an increase in the seizure threshold?

   A Being a female patient
   B Co-administration of antidepressants
   C Co-administration of antipsychotics
   D Increasing age
   E Past history of ECT 5 years ago

CHILD AND ADOLESCENT PSYCHIATRY

91. A 10-year-old boy presented in your clinic with his mother and stepfather. His parents were worried that he was disruptive, defiant and challenging most of the time at home. They wanted to know why he was like this and different from his two siblings. Which of the following is the most relevant risk factor in the development of conduct disorder in children?

   A Drinking during pregnancy
   B Parents with a history of conduct disorder
   C Parents with a forensic history
   D Siblings with a forensic history
   E Urban areas

92. A 13-year-old girl presented with her mother in your clinic with panic attacks and difficulties with breathing. She wanted to know what was wrong with her and also the prevalence of mental disorders in children and adolescents. Which of the following statements is correct?

   A Community prevalence is around 10–15%.
   B Figures of overall prevalence are similar across cultures around the world.
   C Prevalence of moderate-to-severe illnesses is around 6–8%.
   D Proportion of girls with psychiatric diagnoses relative to boys reduces with age.
   E Prevalence of girls with psychiatric disorders is now higher than for in boys.

Questions: MCQs

93. A 16-year-old girl was treated for depression by her GP. She presented in your clinic to discuss the long-term implications of her depression. Which of the following statements about depression in children and adolescents is correct?

    A   Childhood depression is associated with higher rates of depression in adult life.
    B   Depression is less common in boys than in girls up to adolescence.
    C   Point prevalence of depression in adolescents is 7–8%.
    D   Point prevalence of depression in children is 5%.
    E   There is a high rate of recovery but a low rate of relapse in children.

94. A 9-year-old boy attended your clinic with his mother. You would like to discuss parent–child interaction therapy (PCIT), which is a parent training programme, with the mother. Which of the following is a correct statement about PCIT?

    A   The aim of the therapy is to teach a child how to behave appropriately.
    B   It was developed by Fonagy at the University of Florida.
    C   It consists of five phases.
    D   Teaching begins at the clinic and then is gradually taken home.
    E   The therapist takes turns with the parent in playing with the child.

95. A 10-year-old boy with a diagnosis of autism presented with significant irritability, aggression and self-injury. At assessment, no specific underlying cause could be found. After a trial of behaviour management was unsuccessful, it was decided to try a medication. Which of the following medications is considered effective in such a situation?

    A   An antihistamine
    B   Buspirone
    C   Fluoxetine
    D   Methylphenidate
    E   Risperidone

96. A 15-year-old boy was treated for depression by his GP. Unfortunately, his condition got worse. He now presents in your clinic. Which of the following is a first-line treatment?

    A   Dynamic psychotherapy
    B   Family therapy
    C   Fluoxetine
    D   Group therapy
    E   Sertraline

97. A 14-year-old girl who took an overdose of paracetamol and bleach for no apparent reason was brought to the accident and emergency department. She wanted to know why she had tried to harm herself. She also wanted to know how many other children and adolescents self-harm every year. Approximately what proportion of children and adolescents with self-harm present themselves to hospitals in England?

    A   13%
    B   26%
    C   45%
    D   62%
    E   89%

98. A 7-year-old persistently refused to go to school. What is the most common underlying disorder?

    A   Autism
    B   Depression
    C   Panic disorder
    D   Separation anxiety
    E   Specific phobia

99. A 14-year-old severely depressed boy was treated with a combination of CBT and fluoxetine. He was feeling better but could not tolerate fluoxetine's side effects. Which of the following would be the best option to consider as the second line?

   A   Citalopram
   B   Escitalopram
   C   Mirtazapine
   D   Paroxetine
   E   Venlafaxine

100. A 6-year-old boy with autism attended your clinic for a review. His parents would like to know the long-term outcome of their son's condition. Which of the following statements about the prognosis of autism is correct?

   A   Autistic individuals are at an increased risk of developing schizophrenia in adult life.
   B   Autistic children with reasonable speech and normal IQ have good social outcomes in >70% of cases.
   C   Autistic aloofness does not improve with time.
   D   A third of autistic children who do not have useful speech by age 5 will go on to develop it later in life.
   E   About 10% of autistic individuals go through a phase in adolescence when they lose language skills.

101. A 10-year-old girl was diagnosed with a psychiatric condition. Her parents blamed themselves for her condition. You tried to offer some information to them. Which of the following conditions is thought to have a proportionally greater influence of a shared environment than shared genes?

   A   Autism
   B   Conduct disorder
   C   Depression
   D   Hyperkinetic disorder
   E   Schizophrenia

102. A 14-year-old boy with a conduct disorder was brought to your clinic. You discussed his care plan with his parents. Which of the following is considered the best-established approach to manage conduct disorder?

   A   Cognitive-behavioural therapy
   B   Group psychotherapy
   C   Interpersonal psychotherapy
   D   Medication
   E   Parent management training

LEARNING DISABILITY

103. A 39-year-old primipara woman attended your clinic for genetic counselling because she has a family history of an inherited genetic condition. Which of the following genetic conditions is most unlikely to be inherited?

   A   Down's syndrome
   B   Edwards' syndrome
   C   Fragile X syndrome
   D   Klinefelter's syndrome
   E   Turner's syndrome

104. A 30-year-old man with Down's syndrome attended your clinic. He was in a relationship with a 28-year-old woman who also had Down's syndrome. He wanted to know about the chances of having a child. Which of the following statements about fertility in people with Down's syndrome is correct?

   A   Men with Down's syndrome due to non-disjunction have a high incidence of infertility.
   B   Men with mosaic Down's syndrome have a high incidence of infertility.
   C   Women with Down's syndrome due to non-disjunction have a high incidence of infertility.
   D   Women with Down's syndrome due to robertsonian translocation have a high incidence of infertility.
   E   Women with mosaic Down's syndrome have a high incidence of infertility.

105. A 30-year-old man with schizophrenia and learning disability attended your clinic with his support worker for a review. The support worker wanted to know more about the relationship between mental disorders and learning disability. What is the prevalence of psychiatric disorders (excluding behavioural problems) in the learning-disabled population?

   A   5–20%
   B   20–40%
   C   40–50%
   D   50–70%
   E   70–80%

106. A 24-year-old man with a severe learning disability was brought by his support worker to your clinic for a review. The support worker wanted to know more about severe learning disability and its implications for the individual and society. Which of the following statements about the epidemiology of severe intellectual impairment is correct?

   A   Age-specific prevalence varies over time.
   B   Point prevalence is similar between similar birth cohorts in different communities within the UK.
   C   Studies have failed to show a social class gradient consistent with the known social distribution of morbidity and mortality.
   D   There is usually the same proportion of males and females at all ages.
   E   Very different patterns of temporal variation have occurred throughout the developed world.

107. Which of the following is measured by the Life Experiences Checklist?

   A   Disability
   B   Handicap
   C   Impairment
   D   Learning disability
   E   Mental illness

108. Which of the following statements about offending in the learning-disabled (LD) population is correct?

   A   Evidence exists for increased rates of violence in this population.
   B   Learning disability together with obsessive personality features carries a high risk for offending.
   C   Offending is more likely in the severe LD group than the mild-to-moderate group.
   D   Offences are broadly similar to those of offenders without learning disability.
   E   Property offences are committed with excessive forethought.

109. A 7-year-old girl was diagnosed with mild learning disability. She attended your clinic for a review. Her mother had heard about subcultural learning disability. Which of the following statements about subcultural learning disability is correct?

   A   Family members are more likely to have borderline or mild intellectual disability.
   B   It has no relationship with the socioeconomic status of the family in which the child was born.
   C   There are dysmorphic features in children with subcultural learning disability.
   D   There will be impaired adaptive functioning.
   E   There will be a severe degree of learning disability in some family members.

110. An 8-year-old boy studying in year 3 was referred to the learning disability services. Over the past year, he had developed partial blindness, myoclonic jerks and intellectual deterioration. What is the most likely diagnosis?

   A   Batten's disease
   B   Down's syndrome
   C   Parry's disease
   D   Rett's syndrome
   E   Williams' syndrome

111. A 10-year-old boy was diagnosed with dyslexia. He attended your clinic for a review. His father who accompanied him would like to know what deficits the boy is likely to encounter in the future. Which of the following is the primary skill deficit in patients with dyslexia?

   A   Higher linguistics
   B   Impaired rapid automatic naming
   C   Phonological working memory
   D   Single word reading
   E   Syntactic and semantic processing skills

FORENSIC PSYCHIATRY

112. You were asked to assess a prisoner who had been charged with violent offences against members of the public. To complete a comprehensive risk assessment, you decided to use an actuarial tool for violence risk assessment. Which of the following is the most appropriate tool for this purpose?

   A   ESR-20
   B   HCR-20
   C   PCL-R (Hare)
   D   RSVP
   E   SVR-20

113. A 24-year-old man was charged with a criminal offence. However, he pleaded not guilty to the charge. In British law, all offences must be proven to confirm that the accused physically did the act. Which of the following is the most appropriate legal term?

   A   Actus rea
   B   Actus reus
   C   Arcus rea
   D   Mens actus
   E   Mens rea

Questions: MCQs

114. According to current research evidence, what is the percentage of convicted prisoners with psychosis?

    A   4%
    B   6%
    C   8%
    D   10%
    E   15%

115. According to current research evidence, what is the estimated percentage of homicides that are followed by suicide of the perpetrator (homicide–suicide)?

    A   0.5%
    B   1%
    C   2%
    D   5%
    E   10%

116. A 26-year-old man was charged with a violent offence against his girlfriend. However, he pleaded not guilty to the charge because he claimed that it occurred when he was sleepwalking. For his explanation to be plausible, during which stage of sleep does sleepwalking occur?

    A   Rapid eye movement (REM) sleep
    B   Stage 2
    C   Stages 1–2
    D   Stages 2–3
    E   Stages 3–4

117. A 35-year-old man with Asperger's syndrome was charged with a public disorder offence. His solicitors would like to know why he might have committed the alleged offence. They also wanted to know which category of offences individuals with Asperger's syndrome are more likely to commit compared with individuals without it.

    A   Acquisitive
    B   Arson
    C   Drug offences
    D   Fraud
    E   Sexual offences

118. Which of the following statements about Pritchard's criteria to assess fitness to plead in the UK is correct?

    A   It applies criteria at the time of the alleged offence.
    B   Being unfit to plead can result in a trial of facts.
    C   It includes an assessment for fitness to appear in court.
    D   People who are mute are automatically found unfit to plead.
    E   It requires an understanding of previous trials of a similar nature.

119. Which of the following statements about insane automatism in the UK is correct?

    A   It can be caused by an insulinoma.
    B   A defendant has partial control over his actions.
    C   It includes confusional states following anaesthesia.
    D   Intent to harm does not need to be excluded.
    E   The McNaughton rules do not apply.

SUBSTANCE MISUSE/ADDICTIONS

120. A 43-year-old man presented with an alcohol problem. He wanted to know more about his condition including the prognosis. You discussed Jellinek's classification of alcohol problems and considered that he had β alcoholism. Which of the following is a characteristic feature of his condition?

    A   Absence of withdrawal symptoms
    B   Dipsomania
    C   Physical dependence and loss of control
    ·D Polyneuropathy and cirrhosis of the liver
    E   Psychological dependence, drinking to relieve emotional pain

121. According to ICD-10, which of the following statements is correct with regard to criteria for a dependence syndrome?

    A   This involves persisting with a substance with or without evidence of harm.
    B   A physiological withdrawal state should be evident only when substance use has ceased.
    C   A strong desire to take the substance is present every day.
    ,D Three or more manifestations must be present for more than a month.
    E   Tolerance refers to diminished effects with reduced intake of substance.

122. According to ICD-10, which of the following is a character code that may be used to further specify dependence syndrome?

    A   Currently remitting
    B   Currently dependent after partial remission
    C   Currently dependent but receiving treatment
    D   Late remission
    .E Partial remission

123. A 35-year-old man presented with mild alcohol dependence. Which of the following would be the most appropriate psychological intervention for him?

    .A Cognitive–behavioural therapy
    B   Family therapy
    C   Group therapy
    D   Interpersonal therapy
    E   Psychodynamic psychotherapy

124. Which of the following is the proposed mechanism of action of acamprosate in alcohol dependence?

    ˙A GABA agonism
    B   Glutamatergic agonism
    C   NMDA agonist
    D   Noradrenergic antagonism
    E   Serotonin activation

PSYCHOTHERAPY

125. A 23-year-old woman presented with bulimia nervosa in the eating disorders clinic. She would like to know about various treatment options for her condition. Which of the following treatment options for bulimia nervosa has the best evidence base?

    A   Dialectical behavioural therapy
    B   Family therapy

C Self-help
D Serotonin reuptake inhibitors
E Specialised cognitive–behavioural therapy

126. A 37-year-old man with Capgras' syndrome attended your clinic for a review. His care coordinator who would like to learn more about this condition accompanied him. Which of the following statements about Capgras' syndrome is correct?

A It occurs in organic pathological states.
B It involves strangers.
C It is common among individuals with schizophrenia.
D The abnormality is hallucinatory.
E There is a perceived outward change in a person's appearance.

127. You assessed a 45-year-old man with a chronic alcohol problem and morbid jealousy. His partner, who is the mother of his three children, accompanied him. She would like to learn about his condition. Which of the following statements about morbid jealousy is correct?

A It is a common motivation for homicide.
B It is also known as Hamlet's syndrome.
C It is almost always delusional in nature.
D It occurs in women more than men.
E Violence is more often vented on the supposed rival than on the partner.

128. A 25-year-old man complained of seeing roof tiles as a brilliant flaming red. He did not complain of any other psychiatric symptoms. Which of the following terms describes this phenomenon?

A Dysmegalopsia
B Hyperaesthesia
C Hallucination
D Hyperschemazia
E Illusion

129. A 32-year-old man attended your outpatient clinic with his 6-month pregnant wife. He informed you that he could feel his unborn baby's movements in his abdomen. What is this phenomenon known as?

A Autoscopy
B Cotard's syndrome
C Couvade's syndrome
D Irritable bowel syndrome
E Pseudocyesis

130. A depressed 30-year-old woman was assessed and it was considered that she needed to work on her unresolved grief. Her problems were linked to a number of stressors, characteristic patterns of relationships and self-limiting themes that were complex and interactive. Which of the following therapies would be best suited to her needs?

A Cognitive–analytic therapy
B Cognitive–behavioural therapy
C Group therapy
D Long-term individual therapy
E Short-term dynamic therapy

Questions: EMIs

RESEARCH METHODS, STATISTICS, CRITICAL REVIEW AND EVIDENCE-BASED PRACTICE

Theme: Comparison of relationships between different variables

Options for questions: 131–135

A Correlation coefficient
B Kendall's correlational coefficient
C Logistic regression
D Multiple analysis of co-variance
E Multiple analysis of variance
F Multiple linear regression
G Pearson's correlational coefficient
H Proportional Cox's regression
I Simple linear regression
J Spearman's rank correlation coefficient

For each of the following, select the single most appropriate application. Each option may be used once, more than once or not at all.

131. It indicates degree to which two measures are related although it does not explain how.

132. It is a correlational coefficient for two categorical or non-parametrically (non-normally) distributed variables.

133. It is used when the dependent variable is of a dichotomous or binary type (e.g. yes or no), whereas the independent variable can be of any type.

134. It is used with multiple dependent and independent variables.

135. It is used with multiple dependent variables.

Theme: Bias and confounders in research studies

Options for questions: 136–140

A Berksonian bias
B Blinding
C Matching
D Randomisation
E Recall bias
F Restriction
G Stratification
H Systemic sampling

For each of the following situations, select the single most appropriate bias or confounder. Each option may be used once, more than once or not at all.

136. When researchers were evaluating patient's responses, they were kept unaware whether the patients were from the control arm or the experimental arm.

137. A structured interview was used with standardised criteria for diseases and exposures. The information was obtained from more than one source.

138. In a study of schizophrenia, the researchers recruited equal number of cannabis smokers and non-smokers.

139. In a different study of schizophrenia, the researchers excluded all cannabis users from the study and explored variables.

140. In a population-based study of incidence of schizophrenia in the UK, the researchers looked at groups from different income brackets.

GENERAL ADULT PSYCHIATRY

Theme: Psychotic phenomenology in mental disorders

Options for questions: 141–144

A	Auditory hallucination	G	Formal thought disorder
B	Charles Bonnet syndrome	H	Haptic hallucinations
C	Concrete awareness	I	Mania without psychotic features
D	Delirium tremens	J	Synaesthesia
E	Delusional percept	K	Temporal lobe epilepsy (TLE)
F	Depression without psychosis	L	Visceral hallucinations

For each of the following cases, select the single most appropriate description. Each option may be used once, more than once or not at all.

141. A 22-year-old man claimed that he felt, saw, tasted and smelt the music from a trumpet.

142. A 48-year-old man with deteriorating diabetic retinopathy had recently been horrified by visual hallucinations of snakes and green serpents trying to bite him.

143. A 35-year-old Indian man with a history of febrile convulsions was struck on his head by a cricket ball recently. Since then, he has complained of visual hallucinations of seeing his old time friend often talking to him in their local language.

144. A 41-year-old man presented to A&E as experiencing illusions that were frequently associated with hallucinations. They changed so rapidly that it was difficult for him to describe them and he was frightened most of the time.

RESEARCH METHODS, STATISTICS, CRITICAL REVIEW AND EVIDENCE-BASED PRACTICE

Theme: Research methodology and clinical studies

Options for questions: 145–150

A	CAFÉ	G	MTA
B	CATIE	H	POTS
C	CUtLASS 1	I	SOHO
D	DEPRES	J	STAR*D
E	ESEMED	K	TEOSS
F	IPSS	L	TORDIA

For each of the following, select the single most appropriate research study. Each option may be used once, more than once or not at all.

145. First-generation antipsychotic used was perphenazine

146. An observational study conducted in Europe, funded by Eli Lilly, on antipsychotics for schizophrenia

147. Study on depression in Europe funded by SmithKline Beecham Pharmaceuticals

148. Study conducted in six countries across Europe, excluding the UK. Used CIDI to generate questionnaires

149. Study comparing sertraline, CBT and a combination for treatment of OCD in children
150. Study comparing first-generation antipsychotics (FGAs) against second-generation antipsychotics (SGAs) in schizophrenia

Theme: Epidemiological concepts

Options for questions: 151–153

A   Cumulative incidence
B   Life-time prevalence
C   Morbidity rate
D   Point prevalence
E   Period prevalence
F   Standardised mortality rate
G   Standardised mortality ratio

For each of the following cases, select the single most appropriate application. Each option may be used once, more than once or not at all.

151. In your catchment area, you decided to screen all primary schoolchildren for ADHD and found that about 5% of school children had ADHD symptoms.

152. The proportion of participants who had developed a condition within a specified time period.

153. Mortality rate that is adjusted to compensate for age, sex, etc.

Theme: Randomisation methods in research studies

Options for questions: 154–157

A   Minimisation
B   Play the winner
C   Simple randomisation
D   Stratified randomisation
E   Randomised consent method
F   Randomisation permutated blocks

For each of the following cases, select the single most appropriate randomisation method. Each option may be used once, more than once or not at all.

154. In this method, the first participant is allocated by a simple randomisation procedure and then after every subsequent allocation it is based on the success or failure of the immediate predecessor participant.

155. This technique is useful for studies of small size and long duration in which it can ensure that roughly comparable numbers of participants are allocated to study groups at any point in the process.

156. In this method, an eligible population is divided according to a minimum number of important prognostic factors.

157. This method is used in some clinical trials to lessen the effect of some patients refusing to participate.

Theme: Design features of clinical research studies

Options for questions: 158–160

A   Control participants receive a placebo
B   Each group receives a different treatment with both groups being entered at the same time
C   Each participant received both the intervention and the treatment
D   Participants are assessed before and after an intervention

E Results are analysed by comparing groups
F Results are analysed in terms of differences between participant pairs
G Separated by a period of no treatment
H This permits an investigation of the effects of more than one independent variable on a given outcome

For each of the following studies, select TWO most appropriate features. Each option may be used once, more than once or not at all.

158. Cross-over trial

159. Parallel-group comparison

160. Paired comparison

Theme: Randomised control trials

Options for questions: 161–163

A Assumes a poor outcome for drop-outs
B 'Brought forward' data are incorporated into the overall analysis of whichever group they originally belonged to
C Data should be analysed as a unit of randomisation
D Data on all patients entering a trial should be analysed with respect to the groups to which they were originally randomised, regardless of whether or not they received treatment
E Differences in the drop-out rates and the timing of these drop-outs influence the estimation of treatment
F Interventions are directed at groups rather than individual participants
G This may not be appropriate in trials assessing the physiological effects of a drug as opposed to efficacy

For each of the following descriptions, select TWO most appropriate options. Each option may be used once, more than once or not at all.

161. Last data carried forward

162. Intention-to-treat analysis

163. Cluster trials

GENERAL ADULT PSYCHIATRY

Theme: Costs involved in healthcare

Options for questions: 164–166

A Avoiding hospital admission
B Investigations
C Pain and suffering
D Prevention of expensive-to-treat illness
E Social stigma
F Staff salaries
H Value of 'unpaid work'
I Work days lost

For each of the following descriptions, select the TWO most appropriate cost options. Each option may be used once, more than once or not at all.

164. Direct costs

165. Intangible costs

166. Indirect costs

Theme: Medical databases

Options for questions: 167–169

A	Allied and Complementary Medicine Database (AMED)	E	Google Scholar
B	Cumulative Index to Nursing and Allied Health Literature (CINAHL)	F	Health STAR
		G	MEDLINE
		H	PsycINFO
C	Cochrane Library	I	Scopus
D	EMBASE		

For each of the following descriptions, select the single most appropriate database. Each option may be used once, more than once or not at all.

167. It covers health services, hospital administration and health technology assessment.

168. This is a nursing and allied health database.

169. The database of Excerpta Medica focuses on drugs and pharmacology, clinical medicine and other biomedical specialties.

Theme: Architecture of clinical research

Options for questions 170–172

A	Causation can be inferred		qualitative study
B	Examples include controlled clinical trial and economic analyses, systematic reviews and their meta-analyses	E	Generally compare two groups
		F	Generally conducted without a control group
		G	Something is given or done in the experimental group but not in the control group
C	Examples include case-control and cohort studies		
D	Examples include case reports and series, audits, cross-sectional surveys and	H	Suitable for hypothesis generation
		I	Suitable for hypothesis testing

For each of the following studies, select THREE most appropriate descriptions. Each option may be used once, more than once or not at all.

170. Descriptive studies

171. Analytical studies

172. Experimental studies

RESEARCH METHODS, STATISTICS, CRITICAL REVIEW AND EVIDENCE-BASED PRACTICE

Theme: Sources of bias in clinical drug trials

Options for questions: 173–176

A	Double blinding	E	Selection bias
B	Information bias	F	Single blinding
C	Observer bias	G	Triple blinding
D	Recall bias		

For each of the following descriptions, select the single most appropriate source of bias. Each option may be used once, more than once or not at all.

173. It reduces the potential bias of a patient's placebo response.

174. It reduces the doctor's sometimes overzealous desire to find a good new treatment.

175. The analysis of outcomes is conducted by an independent researcher.

176. This is prone to non-blind outcome assessment.

Theme: Measures of disease frequency

Options for questions: 177–180

A   Incidence density
B   Incidence risk
C   Lifetime risk
D   Mortality ratio
E   Period prevalence
F   Point prevalence
G   Standardised mortality ratio

For each of the following cases, select the single most appropriate option. Each option may be used once, more than once or not at all.

177. The number of new cases of the disease over a period of time out of the total population at risk.

178. The number of new cases out of the person-time of observation.

179. The number of individuals with the disease in the population over a period of time.

180. The ratio of observed to expected deaths.

Theme: Sources of error in tests

Options for questions: 181–183

A   Bias towards the centre
B   Extreme responding
C   Halo effect
D   Hawthorne's effect
E   Response set
F   Social acceptability
G   Recollection bias

For each of the following cases, select the single most appropriate source of error. Each option may be used once, more than once or not at all.

181. The participants will always either agree or disagree with the questions and hence the true opinion might not be revealed.

182. The participant chooses answers that might not offend others or the ones that examiners want to know.

183. The participants' responses are altered by the mere presence of the examiner.

GENERAL ADULT PSYCHIATRY

Theme: Frontal lobe brain tumours and respective symptomatology

Options for questions: 184–186

A   Anterior cingulate tumours
B   Bilateral frontal lobe tumours
C   Dorsolateral prefrontal convexity tumours
D   Left frontal lobe tumours

E   Orbitofrontal tumours   F   Tumour of falx

For each of the following cases, select the single most appropriate diagnosis. Each option may be used once, more than once or not at all.

184. Impulsivity with behavioural disinhibition

185. Apathy and lack of spontaneity

186. Akinetic mutism

Theme: Contributions to psychiatry

Options for questions: 187–190

A   Benedict Morel   E   John Cade
B   Eugene Bleuler   F   Karl Ludwig Kahlbaum
C   Emil Kraepelin   G   Phillepe Pinel
D   Jacob Kasanin   H   RD Laing

For each of the following cases, select the single most appropriate person. Each option may be used once, more than once or not at all.

187. Associated with the anti-psychiatry movement

188. Coined the term démence precoce

189. Described catatonia for the first time

190. Discovered the effects of lithium as a mood stabiliser

Theme: Cognitive distortions

Options for questions: 191–193

A   Arbitrary inference   F   Minimisation
B   Catastrophising   G   Overgeneralisation
C   Dichotomous thinking   H   Personalisation
D   Disqualifying the positive   I   Selective abstraction
E   Magical thinking

For each of the following descriptions, select the single most appropriate cognitive distortion. Each option may be used once, more than once or not at all.

191. A 30-year-old, hard-working and sincere employee greeted you and complimented you on your achievements. You said that he was doing it to get a promotion in your company.

192. A 16-year-old girl decided not to ask a girl in her class to join her for shopping because she knew that she would say no.

193. A 14-year-old boy played football for his school. He scored a goal and his team won the match. He told his mother that during the game he tripped and almost let in a goal for the other side. He said that he was rubbish at football and did not wish to play again.

CHILD AND ADOLESCENT PSYCHIATRY

Theme: First-line medication for disorders in children and adolescents

Options for questions: 194–196

A   Acute mania
B   Conduct disorder
C   Mild ADHD without co-morbidity
D   Mild depression
E   Moderate depression
F   Schizophrenia
G   Severe ADHD without co-morbidity
H   Gilles de la Tourette's syndrome
I   Young people with borderline personality disorder

For each of the following drugs, select the single most appropriate diagnosis for which it is indicated. Each option may be used once, more than once or not at all.

194. Fluoxetine

195. Methylphenidate

196. Olanzapine

LEARNING DISABILITY

Theme: Behavioural symptoms associated with learning disability

Options for questions: 197–200

A   Angelman's syndrome
B   Cornelia de Lange's syndrome
C   Down's syndrome
D   Fragile X syndrome
E   Lesch–Nyhan syndrome
F   Prader–Willi syndrome
G   Rett's syndrome
H   Tuberous sclerosis
I   Velocardiofacial syndrome
J   Williams' syndrome

For each of the following cases, select the single most appropriate diagnosis. Each option may be used once, more than once or not at all.

197. Verbal and physical aggression; self-injurious behaviour such as biting lips, inside of the mouth and fingers, thumping of the ears and face, hitting the head against objects; severe learning disability; hypertonia, ataxia and involuntary movements.

198. Abnormalities in speech; cognitive impairment with relatively intact visuospatial skills, reduced short-term memory and greater loss from memory over time; sleep abnormalities; good tempered and cheerful; severe behavioural problems associated with hyperphagia, self-injurious behaviour particularly in the form of incessant spot picking and temper tantrums.

199. Severe or profound learning disability; lack of speech; ataxia; inappropriate bouts of laughter; tongue thrusting; hand flapping and mouthing behaviour.

200. Episodes of low mood; episodes of anxiety with hyperventilation, screaming, self-injury, a frightened expression and general distress precipitated by sudden noises, certain music, strange people or places, changes in routine and excessive environmental activity; self-injurious behaviour associated with abnormal hand movements including biting and chewing of fingers and hands; sleep problems including laughing at night and autistic features.

Answers: MCQs

1. B There should be at least one trained nurse in the recovery area

There should be at least one trained nurse in the treatment area. The ECT team has to be same every week in the clinic. It is the ECT psychiatrist who develops protocol for ECT prescription. There should be at least one person competent in cardiopulmonary resuscitation for every unconscious patient.

2. B An 'ECT rights about consent to treatment' leaflet is provided to detained patients

Consent should be obtained by the referring psychiatrist and checked by the ECT psychiatrist before administering any treatment. ECT information must be provided both verbally and in written form. Explanation on the adverse effects of ECT on cognition must be provided. Capacity assessment must be documented for all patients, including voluntary ('informal') patients.

3. B Increased appetite

The clinical predictors of a response to phototherapy include increased sleep, winter weight gain, carbohydrate craving, afternoon slump in energy and complete remission in the summer. Lack of bright light in winter months is considered a major cause of seasonal affective disorder, and is also known as 'winter blues'. Light entering our eyes stimulates the daily mood rhythm in the brain by hormone production. Although light therapy is a popular treatment, there is no strong evidence to support its long-term benefit.

4. E The intensity of rTMS is usually set as a percentage of the patient's motor threshold

rTMS stands for repetitive transcranial magnetic stimulation. The procedure can be carried out as outpatient and does not need anaesthesia. During the procedure magnetic impulses are delivered in pulses to focussed area of patient's brain. These lead to involuntary twitching of skeletal muscles. Hence the intensity of rTMS pulse waves depending on the patient's motor threshold (MT). MT is defined as the minimum stimulus strength required evoking skeletal muscle twitching at least five times out of ten. Usually the patient does not develop seizures.

5. C Obsessive compulsive disorder

Other indications include anxiety disorders and major depression. Psychosurgery requires informed consent and the approval of an independent review board. The patients must be 20 years or older and have a minimum of 3 years' disease duration with at least 2 years of unremitting symptoms despite active treatment. All patients must fulfil ICD-10 diagnostic criteria. Psychosurgery cannot be performed against the patient's wishes under the Mental Health Act.

6. E The Camberwell Assessment of Need

The other measures include Medical Research Council Needs for Care Assessment, Cardinal Needs Schedule, The Avon Mental Health Measure and the Carers and Users Experience of Services. The Camberwell Assessment of Need assesses 22 domains of health and social need. It records staff and patient views separately without giving primacy to either perspective. It has been translated into 22 languages and is the most widely used needs assessment internationally.

7. A An offence against someone with a mental disorder who is unable to refuse

There are three categories of offence against those with mental disorders.

- Offences against patients who are 'unable to refuse'
- Offences against persons who are vulnerable and at risk of deception though have capacity to consent to sexual activity
- Offences by care worker against patients with mental disorder

The legal definition of mental disorder in the act from the Crown Prosecution Service (2005) is the same as in the Mental Health Act 1983 (amended 2007).

8. D Patient should stop driving for at least 6 months and inform the DVLA as this is an isolated alcohol-related seizure

DVLA issues guidance to medical practitioners about the advice they should offer to patients. These are updated every six months and are freely available at www.dft.gov.uk/dvla/medical/ataglance.aspx. The guidelines related to alcohol or substance misuse mention that a person should stop driving immediately and inform DVLA, if he suffers from harmful use of alcohol or alcohol dependence. In this scenario, the patient has suffered an isolated alcohol-related seizure. Hence, he should stop driving and inform DVLA. His driving license would be revoked by DVLA for a period of at least 6 months. If he suffers recurrent seizures related to alcohol misuse, then epilepsy guidance related to driving should be followed.

9. C Inpatient suicide by hanging using a non-collapsible curtain rail

Never events are defined as 'serious, largely preventable patient safety incidents'. The Department of Health has identified certain health care related events as 'never events'. Occurrences of these events have serious implications for the service providers as these can be prevented by appropriate measures. Only one mental health-related incident is classified as a never event: death or serious harm to a mentally ill inpatient as a result of a suicide attempt using non-collapsible curtain or shower rails. This led to the use of collapsible rails in inpatient mental health wards in England and a reduction in inpatient suicide rates.

10. D 0.95

The experimental event rate (EER) is the event rate in the experimental, active or exposed group of patients. It is calculated by dividing the number of patients experiencing an event by the total number of patients:

EER: 190/200 = 0.95.

11. C 0.6

Clinical drug trials measure outcomes in a number of ways. First, and arguably the least clinically useful, the outcome measure is a symptoms rating scale – a continuous measure. From this, an effect size can be calculated. Second, and clinically most useful, it is a dichotomous measure such as admission or readmission, dead or alive, relapses or non-relapses. In these studies, it is possible to obtain the control event rate (CER). This is simply the frequency of the event in question in the control group; it is calculated by dividing the number of control participants experiencing an event by the total number of control participants:

CER: 120/200 = 0.6.

12. C *0.35*

The absolute benefit increase (ABI) is the absolute numerical difference between the rates of good outcomes between the experimental and control groups in a clinical study. The ABI is calculated from the difference between experimental and control event rates:

ABI = EER − CER = 0.95 − 0.6 = 0.35.

13. B *3*

Usually the NNT is rounded off to the whole number, so the correct answer would be 3. The NNT measures the efficacy of a treatment. It is calculated from the reciprocal of the absolute benefit increase or absolute risk reduction. An NNT value <10 is regarded as clinically significant:

NNT = 1/CER − EER

= 1/0.35

= 2.85.

14. D Type 1 error

This occurs when a difference is found between two groups, although in fact there is no difference (false positive) and a null hypothesis is rejected. In other words, it is the false rejection of a null hypothesis when there is no true difference. It may happen as a result of bias or confounders. The probability of making a type 1 error is equal to the *p* value and is denoted by α. The power is the probability of demonstrating a significant difference between groups, where one exists. The standard deviation is a standardised measure of data dispersion. It is the spread of all observations around the mean and is calculated as the square root of the variance. The probability is the likelihood of any event occurring relative to a different number of possibilities.

15. E Type 2 error

This happens when the null hypothesis is accepted but is not actually true – when there is a small sample size and/or large variance. In other words, a type 2 error is the false acceptance of a null hypothesis when there is a true difference. The power of study is the probability of rejecting the null hypothesis when a true difference exists. Accuracy refers to the degree to which each research project's methodology, instruments and tools are related to each other. It also measures whether research tools have been selected appropriately and whether the research methodology suits the hypothesis under investigation.

16. C Standard deviation

This is the average distance of observations from their mean. It is calculated by squaring each variation or deviation from the mean in a group of scores, then adding the squared deviations; this is then divided by the number of scores in the group minus 1, and the square root of the result is determined:

$SD = \sqrt{\Sigma(x - x^-)^2 \div n - 1}$,

where x is the individual values, x^- the mean and n the total number of observations. Skewedness is a departure from the normal distribution. When the right-hand tail is extended, it is called a positive skew, and when the left-hand tail is extended a negative skew. The standard error is a measure of the uncertainty of a point estimate. It is in fact the spread or the SD of the sample mean. Confidence intervals are derived from the standard error.

17. E 99.7%

A normal distribution is also known as gaussian or bell shaped, and theoretically the mean, median and mode are equal. Approximately 68% of the population scores fall within first standard deviation of the mean, approximately 95% within 2 SDs and 99.7% within 3 SDs. Normally distributed data enable researchers to use parametric statistical tests, which have greater power than non-parametric tests. When variables follow a certain frequency over time or space, it is known as a Poisson distribution. When the result of a research study is a proportion, it is called a binomial distribution. In a t distribution, the continuous variable is measured and its mean difference between two groups estimated.

18. D Power

This is the ability to detect a significant difference between groups. It is also a measure of the strength of the relationship between two variables. The larger the sample size, the more power a researcher has to detect the difference. The power is also defined as the probability of rejecting the null hypothesis when a true difference exists. The type 1 error is α and the type 2 error β. The effect size is the difference between two means, which is divided by the standard deviation in controls.

19. A Mann–Whitney U test

In parametric tests, comparing two groups independently, the student's independent *t*-test is used and, for paired groups, the student's paired *t*-test. For comparing more than two groups, analysis of variance (ANOVA) is used. In non-parametric studies, comparing two unpaired and paired groups, the Mann–Whitney U test and Wilcoxon's rank sum test are used, respectively. The Kruskal–Wallis analysis of variance is used for comparing more than two groups in non-parametric studies. In binary statistics, the χ^2 and McNemar's tests are used for comparing unpaired and paired data, respectively. The χ^2 test is used to compare more than two groups in binary statistical tests.

20. A Analysis of variance (ANOVA)

Comparing more than two groups in parametric, non-parametric and binary statistical tests, the ANOVA, Kruskall–Wallis ANOVA and χ^2 test are used, respectively.

21. A ≥0.04

Probability is the chance of a type 1 error occurring. If the probability of making a type 1 error is equal to the p value then it is expressed as α. If α = 0.05, this means that there is only a 5% chance of erroneously rejecting the null hypothesis.

22. D −1 to + 1

The linear regression is the degree of relationship between two continuous, normally distributed variables that can be assessed using a linear correlation coefficient that ranges between −1 and

+1. This is a parametric correlation coefficient (Pearson's 'r') and it can be plotted as a straight line. A correlation coefficient of 1 would indicate perfect positive correlation (i.e. both values rise together), whereas a value of −1 indicates perfect negative correlation. A correlation coefficient of 0 indicates that there is no relationship between the two variables.

23. B 4 ± 0.68

The confidence interval (CI) or confidence limit is an important measure of dispersion of data. Its properties fill the gap between analytical and descriptive statistics. It is defined as the range within which the true measure of the dispersion of data lies with a specific degree of certainty. One can be 95% certain that the true value of a measure such as a mean lies within a 95% confidence interval or two confidence limits of the estimate:

$SE = SD \div \sqrt{n} = 1.4 \div \sqrt{16} = 1.4 \div 4 = 0.35$

The 95% CI ≈ mean ± 1.96 × SE

≈ 4 ± 1.96 × 0.35

≈ 4 ± 0.686

≈ 3.314 – 4.686

24. A Face validity

This measures the subjective assessment that the item appears to measure the desired quality. The criterion validity is the measure consistent with what we already know (gold standard) and what we expect. The concurrent validity is the extent to which the new measure relates to a different scale measuring something similar. The construct or predictive validity is the measure related to other variables as required by the theory. The convergent validity measures the degree of agreement between the measurements made using two different approaches, which are supposed to measure the same type of traits. The divergent validity measures the results obtained by an instrument that do not correlate too strongly with measurements of similar but distinct traits. It is useful to establish the construct validity of a construct/concept in a study by assessing whether it is different from other constructs in the proposed study.

25. B Construct validity

The predictive validity measures the extent to which a new measure predicts the outcome accurately. The convergent validity measures the degree of agreement between the measurements using two different approaches, which are supposed to measure the same type of traits. It therefore helps to establish the construct validity of a construct/concept in a study. The construct validity shows whether the findings gel with the theory. The content validity is the subjective assessment involved in the instrument sampling all the important contents of the attribute that is being measured.

26. B Internal consistency

The strength of the quantitative approach lies in its reliability. Internal consistency measures whether the score of the items correlates with the scores of all other items of the same construct. For internal consistency, a common approach is to calculate Cronbach's α for continuous data. It is an average of all correlations between various items. It gives an estimate of the reliability of a psychometric test. Cronbach's α (alpha aign) can be regarded as an extension of the Kuder–Richardson formula 20, which is used for dichotomous items. It is widely used in business, nursing, social sciences such as anthropology, archaeology, criminology, psychology, sociology, etc. The test–re-test or interrater reliability, measured at two different times with no treatment in between, should yield the same result. Its typical indices are k. The interobserver reliability measures the agreement among interviewers who are rating the same information. The intraclass correlation coefficient is used in continuous data, and is useful when there is disagreement among various assessors in a research study.

27. A Berkson's bias

This is a false association discovered through a survey of an unrepresentative sample. It is a subtype of sampling bias, also called admission bias. It is used in descriptive research and case–control studies. Researchers or participants can bring in the selection bias. The referral from a general practitioner to secondary care increases the concentration of rare exposures and severe diseases, which is an example of a 'referral filter bias'. The exclusion of co-morbidity introduces a 'diagnostic purity bias' and makes the sample unrepresentative. Recruiting a member of an organisation may introduce a membership bias. Comparison of a new treatment in a current series of patients with an old treatment in a previous series of patients may be subject to historical control bias. When two groups of participants are enrolled in different ways and differ significantly as a result, it leads to an 'ascertainment bias'.

28. C Interobserver reliability

This measures the agreement among raters who are rating the same information. Cronbach's α is associated with internal consistency; k covers many similar measures of agreement in categorical data. It is a measure of diagnostic agreement among raters, which is corrected for the agreement expected by chance.

29. D Hawthorne's effect

This is a non-specific effect caused by the participants' knowledge that they are taking part in the study. The halo effect is the tendency of a rater to overestimate a participant's response based on prior assumptions. People might try to please the experimenter as a goal and this may be called a demand effect. When a simulated medical intervention is given to the patient that may lead to perceived or actual improvement in a medical condition it is known as a placebo effect. The domino effect is defined as a chain reaction when a small change leads to another small change, and then a series of changes in a linear sequence. It can be described as a mechanical effect and is analogous to falling rows of dominos. Practically, it refers to a sequence of events linked to each other where time between successive events is relatively short. The domino effect can be considered both literally and metaphorically.

30. D Prevalence–incidence bias

This is a type of experimenter's bias, also known a as Neyman's bias and selective survival bias. It can occur in case–control and cross-sectional studies. In case–control studies, it is attributed to selective survival among the prevalent cases, but excludes mild, clinically resolved or fatal cases from the case group. Information bias is the general difficulty in assessing past exposures retrospectively. It arises as a result of misclassification of exposure to an agent being studied or misclassification of the disease or its outcome in a study. Publication bias refers to the phenomenon by which studies with positive results are more likely and studies with negative results less likely to be published. As the leading medical journals encourage reporting negative studies, it is becoming less of a problem. It can be evaluated using funnel plots and Galbraith's plots. Confounding bias is an error in the interpretation that could be a correct finding.

31. A Clinical Practice Guidelines

Critically appraised databases are Clinical Practice Guidelines, Clinical Evidence, Evidence-Based Medicine and Evidence-Based Mental Health. They are systematically evaluated and developed statements supporting clinicians and patients to make clinical decisions for special circumstances. They give explicit grade recommendations according to the quality of reviewed evidence.

Biological Abstracts, Cinahl, Cochrane library, EMBASE, PsycINFO and PubMed are electronic databases. There is little quality control and each database probably covers about 40% of the literature on a particular topic.

32. A Affective disorders

According to the current evidence omega-3 essential fatty acids are found to be beneficial in the prevention and/or treatment of unipolar or bipolar depression together with standard pharmacological treatment. The evidence for the treatment benefits for schizophrenia is less significant. They are also useful in various disorders that benefit from fatty acid supplementation, especially omega-3 fatty acids, e.g. rheumatoid arthritis. They provide protective benefit in heart disease and sudden cardiac death. They play a crucial role in brain functions, and normal growth and development, and they reduce inflammation. The main benefits of omega-3 essential fatty acids come from eicosapentaenoic acid (EPA) and docosahexaenoic acid (DHA), which are found in cold water fish, e.g. salmon, sardines, tuna.

33. B If x = 0.01, there is a probability of 1% that the null hypothesis is wrongly rejected.

The null hypothesis states that there is no difference or association between two or more groups of participants in a research study. In statistical terms, it is about disproving the null hypothesis rather than proving it. The factor x is the probability of a type 1 error. It is used to set the threshold for statistical significance, often arbitrarily as $p = 0.01 – 0.05$ ($x = 1–5\%$), meaning that, if $x = 0.01$, there is a 1 in 100 or 1% chance that the true hypothesis is wrongly rejected.

34. A Mean > median

The mean is the average value derived by adding all the measurements, and then dividing the total by the number of measurements. The median is the middle value that divides the distribution into two equal halves. The mode is the most frequently occurring value in a data-set. When many observations are significantly higher than the median, we can assume that the mean of the distribution might be greater than the median. This translates to a positively skewed distribution.

35. A Allocation concealment

This refers to the process used to prevent prior knowledge of assignment before an allocation of participants has been completed. It seeks to prevent selection bias and also prevents the allocation sequence before and up to the assignment. Therefore, the investigators will not know the nature of the assignment of subsequent participants who enter the randomisation. To be properly randomised in a clinical trial, it should use a randomisation schedule that is not predictable. Blinding seeks to prevent ascertainment bias and protects the sequence after allocation. Matching refers to allocating the participants to treatment groups according to set criteria to achieve uniform groups across the board. Blinding and masking are interchangeable terms and they refer to the fact that the participants and/or investigators are unaware of the study treatment.

36. C Q statistics

In a meta-analysis, the results of different studies are combined because individual studies are often too small to yield reliable treatment effects. Although similar studies are included in the meta-analysis, there is a possibility that each study differs from all the others just by chance. Sometimes, the differences can be due to foreseeable factors such as dose of drugs tested, mean

Answers: MCQs

age of the study population, different rating scales, etc. To measure whether this heterogeneity is more than random (expected), it is necessary to conduct certain tests of heterogeneity. These include Q statistics (e.g. χ^2 test), which tests the null hypothesis of homogeneity. A χ^2 test measures the amount of variability due to heterogeneity. Galbraith's plot and the l'Abbé plot are pictorial representations of heterogeneity. The paired Student's t statistic is useful for examining differences in the means of two populations consisting of independent samples, continuous data or at least interval and normally distributed data with equal variances. Stratification is the process of allocating participants in a study population to homogeneous groups before sampling takes place.

37. B Clinical significance of the results

Randomised controlled trials are conducted under strict protocols, which include inclusion and exclusion criteria. The study population (highly homogeneous) may not represent the general population, which is often encountered in clinical practice. Therefore, there is poor generalisability of research findings to daily clinical work.

38. A Taking amphetamines during pregnancy does not increase the risk of ADHD in the child.

If the psychiatric trainee wants to prove that pregnant mothers taking amphetamines increase the risk of ADHD in their offspring, it is necessary to consider the null hypothesis. It is best to assume that maternal consumption of amphetamines does not increase the risk of ADHD and then proceed to disprove it. The converse of the null hypothesis is known as the alternative hypothesis.

39. B Identifying a suitable control group

In a cohort study, there is no need to randomise the participants, so there is no need to conceal allocation. It is often most difficult to identify a reasonable control group that lacks the exposure of interest of the study. Using valid instruments and reasonable follow-up, it is easy to analyse the findings.

40. B 2.5

In the above study, the control event rate (CER) is 20%. The experiment event rate (EER) is 70%.

The absolute rate reduction (ARR) is the difference between the two event rates, i.e. 70 − 20 = 50%

The relative risk reduction (RRR) = 50/20 = 2.5. In other words, the ARR is the absolute numerical difference between the rates of adverse outcomes between the study and the control samples.

The RRR, i.e. the relative benefit increase, is calculated as follows:

RRR = ARR.

41. A 2

Two patients must be treated with aripiprazole to have one additional response. The NNT can be calculated from the absolute risk reduction (ARR):

NNT = 1/ARR = 1/0.5 = 2.

42. B 9.3

The odds ratio refers to comparison of the odds of an event happening in a study group with that happening in another group, e.g. a control group. To calculate the odds ratio, it will be useful to construct a 2 × 2 table. As per protocol, analysis is used, except that those patients who completed the study will be included in the analysis (**Table 1.2**).

Table 1.2 A 2 × 2 table

Study arm	Response	No response	Total
Aripiprazole	70 (a)	30 (b)	100
Placebo	20 (c)	80 (d)	100

The odds ratio is calculated using the cross-product ratio
$ad/bc = (70 \times 80)/(30 \times 20) = 5600/600 = 9.3$.

43. E The direction of the effect cannot be determined.

Cross-sectional studies simultaneously ascertain the presence or absence of both disease and an exposure at a particular point in time. They are effectively studies of prevalence or frequency of disease. They cannot reliably distinguish cause and effect. The direction of the effect cannot be determined because the risk and outcome are being studied at the same time. The other factors are less of a problem or similar in difficulty for other study designs as well.

44. C Systematic reviews of RCTs are above systematic reviews of cohort studies.

The evidence must contain an explicit and reproducible method for weighing the results according to quality and precision. In formulating clinical practice guidelines, a well-conducted meta-analysis with little or no heterogeneity of RCTs is accepted as the highest recommendation.

Hierarchy of evidence for clinical practice guideline recommendation

Level of evidence clinical studies

IA	Systematic reviews and meta-analyses of RCTs
IB	RCTs
IIA	Well-designed non-RCTs
IIB	Other well-designed quasi-experimental studies
III	Evidence from well-designed non-experimental studies
IV	Evidence from expert committee reports and respected authorities

45. A Individual RCTs

A randomised treatment trial of two types of family interventions reported on anorexia nervosa. The study included 'conjoint family therapy' (CFT) and 'separated family therapy' (SFT). A stratified design was used to control for levels of critical comments using the expressed emotion index. The researchers undertook both forms of therapies with separate supervisors. Marked symptomatic improvement was noticed in the SFT group and psychological change in the CFT group.

46. A Individuals show improvement because they are aware of their participation in research.

Individuals improve just because they are being studied. Smaller sample sizes giving false-positive results are called type 2 errors. The other answers are not described by any particular phenomenon.

Answers: MCQs

47. A It stops the selection biases from creeping back into the study.

Intention-to-treat analysis helps to reduce bias. In interventional studies, there are possibilities of participants dropping out or moving from one arm to another for various reasons. It takes into account all these participants and analyses them based on the original study protocol. It prevents selection biases from creeping back into the study and helps to avoid overestimating the benefits of treatment.

48. D Replication studies on a different population help to add weight to the findings.

Such studies in different populations and different parts of the country add weight to the original findings. Ethical approval would still be required and may not be any easier to get than for an original study. Although it may be advantageous, it is not mandatory to use exactly the same methods as the original study. There is a marked publication bias because studies with positive results tend to be reported and published more often than those with negative results. In studies using humans we can never be certain about how representative the sample was. It is therefore always important to repeat studies with different samples in different parts of a country or the world.

49. C Research with positive results has a higher chance of being published.

Publication bias is implied when positive studies tend to be reported and published more often than negative ones. It is not uncommon to find a similar study design being carried out at different centres, because work done with negative results hardly ever gets published. This is not deliberate suppression of data, but an understandable desire for researchers and journals to publish positive findings.

50. D It is also known as a dichotomous variable.

A variable is something that we measure, manipulate and control in an experiment. There are different ways of describing and differentiating variables. A binary variable takes only two possible values and helps to describe binary data with only two mutually exclusive categories. A variable that can take any value within a limited range is called a continuous variable. A variable can be converted into a binary variable, e.g. by defining a cut-off. A dependent variable is a variable that is dependent on the independent variable – also called an outcome variable. An independent variable is a variable that is being examined in an experiment to identify its effect on the dependent variable – also called an experimental or predictor variable. In non-experimental research, the researchers do not manipulate the independent variable because it might be unethical or impractical to do so.

51. A It was conducted in three academic centres between 1997 and 2002.

POTS was conducted in three academic centres across the USA. The main objectives were to evaluate the efficacy of cognitive–behavioural therapy (CBT) alone, sertraline alone, and CBT and sertraline combined as an initial treatment for children and adolescents with obsessive–compulsive disorder (OCD). The duration of treatment was 12 weeks and the participants were recruited between September 1997 and December 2002. The findings of the study suggested that children and adolescents should start treatment with a combination of CBT plus an SSRI or CBT alone.

52. A All-cause discontinuation was the primary outcome measure.

Compared with other antipsychotics, quetiapine was less potent in treating the illness. Of the three antipsychotics compared, risperidone was associated with the smallest elevations in fasting triglyceride and cholesterol levels. The overall PANSS scores were comparable in all three arms; however, greater reduction in a positive symptom subscale was persistently seen in the olanzapine arm. Safety and tolerability were a secondary measure.

53. B Cost Utility of the Latest Antipsychotics in Schizophrenia Study 1

CUtLASS 1 stands for Cost Utility of the Latest Antipsychotic Drugs in Schizophrenia Study 1. It was a randomised controlled trial of the effect on quality of life of second- versus first-generation antipsychotic drugs used to manage schizophrenia. It was conducted by the Institute of Psychiatry in London and was funded by the NHS.

54. D One of the outcome measures included scores of quality-of-life scales.

Outcome measures included quality-of-life scores, symptoms, adverse effects, participant satisfaction and costs of care. Clozapine was considered in CUtLASS 2, not in this study. Depot preparations of the first-generation antipsychotics were taken into account. Some 227 participants from 14 community psychiatric services in the NHS were randomised.

55. C Qualitative research

The best way to achieve a deeper understanding of a particular clinical issue is through qualitative studies. They help to generate ideas, opinions and hypotheses. If they are conducted well, they offer insight and are valid. They can also inform and improve the quality of quantitative research. However, they are prone to researchers' bias and lack reliability if only one researcher was involved. They can illuminate complex issues. If we want to find out the incidence or check the cause-and-effect hypothesis for an exposure and outcome, we can use case–control and cohort studies, which are mainly observational studies. To find out which treatment or intervention is better in a population, we should use RCTs. Cross-sectional studies are helpful in finding out the prevalence.

56. B Cost-effectiveness analysis

This is a form of economic analysis that compares the cost of an organised treatment/intervention or activity with its effectiveness, measured in terms of natural health outcomes, e.g. life-years gained. It means that, if there is more than one strategy with similar results, cost-effective analysis is used to identify the most cost-effective strategy of the lot. It is usually expressed as the cost per health outcome, e.g. the amount earned by preventing cases of polio through use of the vaccine compared with the cost of polio vaccine itself.

57. B External validity

This term is used to describe the quality of a systematic review. It refers to the degree to which conclusions of one study would hold together different people in different places and at different times. Assigning weight to trials in a systematic review involves looking at methodological quality, precision and external validity, as well as other features.

58. B Catatonia

The Bush–Francis rating scale is used to assess catatonia. It is available as a 23-item scale as well as a shorter version, consisting of 14 items. The Simpson–Angus scale and abnormal involuntary movements scale (AIMS) are useful in assessing extrapyramidal side effects. Catatonia is characterised by marked psychomotor retardation, which may be accompanied by motoric immobility or excessive motor activity, mutism, excessive negativism, echolalia, echopraxia or abnormal voluntary movements. Malignant catatonia (replacing the term 'lethal catatonia') is characterised by autonomic instability and hyperthermia. Catatonia is usually associated with schizophrenia and mood disorders, and less frequently with neurological, endocrine and metabolic disorders, infections, and drug withdrawal and toxicity. Most catatonic patients respond to benzodiazepine (especially lorazepam) within 3–7 days. ECT is helpful in catatonia presenting in schizophrenia and mood disorders.

59. B Depressive disorder with psychotic symptoms

Depressive mood preceded the psychotic symptoms. In this case, the psychotic symptoms are mood congruent and not of definite schizophrenic type (ICD-10 criteria a–d of schizophrenia). Therefore, this is more likely to be a depressive episode with psychosis. The patient does not fulfil the ICD-10 criteria for schizophrenia, post-schizophrenic depression or schizoaffective disorder. There is no evidence of mania.

60. D Prisoners awaiting trial

Ganser's syndrome is characterised by sudden, abrupt ending, 'approximate answers' (Ganser's symptom, *vorbeireden*), clouding of consciousness and amnesia of the episode, auditory and visual hallucinations or pseudo-hallucinations, and dissociative symptoms. In the choice of answers, the patient appears deliberately to pass over the indicated correct answer to select a false one, which any child could recognise as such. It is a rare phenomenon and is more likely to be seen in those prisoners who are awaiting trial. It has been thought of as schizophrenia, an acute psychotic reaction or factitious/simulated psychosis. It is treated as an acute schizophrenic episode.

61. B Impaired glucose tolerance

In anorexia nervosa, cortisol-releasing hormone, cortisol, growth hormone and reverse triiodothyronine (T_3) levels are increased whereas LH, follicle-stimulating hormone (FSH), somatomedin C, T_3 and C-peptide are decreased. Anorexia nervosa is also associated with hypokalaemic and hypochloraemic alkalosis caused by vomiting. Insulin release is delayed and glucose tolerance impaired. It is important to differentiate anorexia nervosa from weight loss due to other causes and the above changes will help.

62. D Family therapy

This scenario appears to be a case of high expressed emotions within the family environment. Family therapy including psychoeducation of family members would be helpful. CBT will not be of any help in this scenario because there are no cognitive distortions and the patient is already making good progress. For the same reasons, the community treatment order under the Mental Health Act is also not indicated because the patient has engaged with the services. Interpersonal therapy is less likely to be helpful, and is mainly indicated in depression. Counselling could be helpful if family therapy is not available.

63. A Disorganised schizophrenia

This is characterised by disorganised speech, disorganised behaviour, and flat or inappropriate affect. It is classified in DSM-IV but not in ICD-10. DSM-IV includes paranoid, disorganised, catatonic, undifferentiated and residual subtypes.

ICD-10 also includes paranoid, catatonic and simple schizophrenia subtypes. Post-schizophrenic depression is characterised by the presence of significant depressive symptoms of at least 2 weeks' duration in the aftermath of schizophrenia, but in the presence of some schizophrenic symptoms, which do not dominate the clinical picture.

64. E Simple schizophrenia

This is characterised by insidious and progressive deterioration for at least 1 year when the patient is unable to meet the demands of society and declines in total performance. Negative symptoms appear without any prior psychotic symptoms. Delusions and hallucinations are not evident in these patients. Asperger's syndrome, autism and schizoid personality disorder would be present from childhood and continue into adulthood. Catatonic schizophrenia is dominated by psychomotor disturbances that alternate between stupor and hyperkinesia or automatic obedience and negativism.

65. D Family history of depression

Prognostic factors were carefully identified by Valliant and others for patients with schizophrenia before operational definitions were used. Valliant's predictors of a good prognosis in schizophrenia are less central to the disorder, and include: an acute onset of illness, the presence of a stressful precipitating event, a family history of depressive illness, prominent affective symptoms, an absence of family history of schizophrenia or schizoid premorbid personality traits, and confusion or perplexity. Overall, the outcome seems to be determined more by the circumstances under which the illness develops and the premorbid personality than by the clinical features of the illness. Various studies have observed that, of patients with first-episode schizophrenia, 50% improve, 20% experience no further episode, 40% obtain employment/higher education and 20% live independently.

66. C A fugue state is usually associated with a period of wandering, for which there is a subsequent amnesic gap on recovery.

The fugue state is a syndrome in which there is a sudden loss of all autobiographical memories and knowledge of personal identity, usually associated with a period of wandering, for which there is a subsequent amnesic gap on recovery. Fugue states differ from transient global amnesia or transient epileptic amnesia in that the person does not know whom he or she is. Fugue states are almost always preceded by a severe precipitating stress. Depressed mood is also an extremely common antecedent for a psychogenic fugue state.

67. B It is found more commonly *post mortem* in people with alcohol problems than it is diagnosed in life.

Korsakoff's syndrome is caused by thiamine deficiency. It can arise due to medical conditions. However, the most common cause is chronic and persistent alcohol misuse. This leads to retrograde amnesia and confabulation. In many patients with atypical symptoms, the clinical diagnosis could be easily missed. The confirmation is made *post mortem*, when damage to mammillary bodies and anterior thalamic nuclei is shown.

68. A Herpes encephalitis can give rise to a severe form of amnesic syndrome.

Most cases are said to be due to primary infections, although there may be a history of a preceding 'cold sore' on the lips. Usually there is a fairly abrupt onset of acute fever, headache and nausea. There may be behavioural changes and seizures can occur. The fully developed clinical neuropathological and neuroimaging studies show that there is extensive bilateral temporal lobe damage.

69. A Absence of voluntary control on facial expressions

Pathological laughter and crying (PLC) is defined as uncontrollable laughter, crying or both in the absence of an associated affect. It is also known as a pseudo-bulbar affect or emotional incontinence. It is a primary disorder of emotional expression and not a disorder of feelings. It occurs due to non-specific stimuli and there is no corresponding mood change. In fact, it is associated with feelings of happiness and sadness. PLC is probably caused by loss of the voluntary inhibition of the laughter and crying centre, presumably located in the upper brain stem. It has been noted in a variety of neurological conditions, e.g. galactic epilepsy, multiple sclerosis, pseudo-bulbar palsy, cerebellopontine tumours, trigeminal neuralgia and petroclival meningioma. Amitriptyline 75 mg has been found to be effective. Fluoxetine, sertraline, amantadine or levodopa can also be used.

70. A The patient can present with subcortical dementia.

Cognitive impairment is likely to be subcortical dementia because multiple sclerosis involves mainly the white matter. Mania can occur as a part of the physical disorder or secondary to medication. The patients who have a premorbid or family history of affective disorders are at a higher risk of hypomania when treated with steroids. Hence, in this case caution should be exercised. Early onset of illness is associated with increased risk of suicide. Lifetime prevalence of depression is anywhere from 25% to 50%. The co-occurrence of psychosis and multiple sclerosis is not that common.

71. A Chronic fatigue syndrome

The US Centers for Disease Control and Prevention (CDC) criterion for chronic fatigue syndrome is: new onset of severe unexplained fatigue lasting for more than 6 months that is neither related to exertion nor relieved on rest. For the patient this is a functional impairment. In addition, the patient presents with at least four of symptoms such as impaired memory, concentration, sore throat, tender lymph nodes, pain in the joints and muscles, headaches, poorly refreshing sleep and post-exertional malaise for more than 24 hours. Evidence continues to mount to suggest that this syndrome is a discrete post-infectious entity and not simply a variant or disguised mood or anxiety disorder.

72. C Genetic constitution increasing vulnerability to schizophrenia

Among the predictors of schizophrenia, the most interesting concept is schizotaxia, which is used to describe the genetic vulnerability to schizophrenia. It presents as an aggregation of subtle symptoms of brain dysfunction expressed, in part, as negative symptoms, neuropsychological deficits, including working memory/attention problems, problems in long-term memory and concept formation/abstraction, but not as a psychosis. This syndrome is qualitatively similar, although less severe, not fulfilling the criteria for schizophrenia. A study suggested that the symptoms of schizotaxia occur in 20–50% of adult relatives of patients diagnosed with schizophrenia, although genetic liability to develop schizophrenia does not inevitably lead to schizotypal personality disorder, schizoid personality disorder or schizophrenia.

73. B Epilepsy–parasomnias

These sleep disorders are a category of sleep disorders that occur at various stages of sleep. They consist of abnormal and unusual movements, behaviours, emotions, perceptions and dreams. They are classified into two major types: non-rapid eye movement (NREM) parasomnias and rapid eye movement (REM) parasomnias. NREM parasomnias include sleep walking/somnambulism, night terrors, bruxism and restless legs syndrome. REM parasomnias include REM sleep behaviour disorder, recurrent isolated sleep paralysis and cathrenia, which consists of breathholding and expiratory groaning during sleep. The following are the correct associations for the other disorders:

- Dementia–sun downing
- Huntington's disease–frequent awakening
- Kleine-Levin syndrome–hypersomnia
- Parkinsonism–frequent awakening, disturbed circadian rhythm.

74. A Delusions involving the skin

Somatic delusions may present with a delusional belief of skin infestation, in which the patients believe that they have organisms/parasites (usually worm like) crawling over or into the skin/nails. Occasionally they may believe that the bodies are inanimate, similar to seeds. The 'match box' or 'pill box' sign is seen in delusions involving skin where a patient comes up with a small container that has 'insect corpses' or 'eggs', which are usually skin scrapings, dry mucus or possibly pieces of lint.

75. D Overall, the best-attested treatment result refers to somatic subtype.

After starting therapy with an antipsychotic, it takes about 2 weeks before the delusional system starts to ameliorate. If the medication is stopped, the delusions return within days or weeks. Recovery is often good but slow and the illness may continue for a very long time. The patients may need to continue with medication on a long-term basis. The maintenance dose is usually very small. Overall the best-attested treatment result refers to somatic subtype and there is virtually no literature on the grandiose type.

76. E Pseudo-dementia

EEG may aid the differentiation between degenerative brain disease and depressive pseudo dementia. In EEG, there are four components: δ (<4 Hz), θ (4–7 Hz), α (8–13 Hz) and β (>13 Hz) wave. Pronounced flattening of the EEG may raise the possibility of Huntington's disease. Creutzfeldt–Jakob disease has repetitive spike discharge or triphasic sharp wave complexes. In the early stages of Alzheimer's disease, the EEG is nearly always non-specifically abnormal. However, in frontotemporal degenerations, the EEG remains unaffected. In presenile Alzheimer's disease, α waves disappear and show irregular θ waves with superimposed runs of δ waves.

77. D Personality change and incongruous behaviour

The most common psychiatric presentation in Wilson's disease is personality change, which is found in 25% of patients. In another 25% incongruous behaviour is noticed and is usually the reason for referral. Mild cognitive impairment is suspected in around 25%, depression in 21%, psychosis in 2% and disorientation in 7%, irritability in 18% and aggression in 14%. Wilson's disease is also called hepatolenticular degeneration. It is an autosomal recessive disorder in which copper builds up in the body, especially the liver and brain. The faulty gene ATP7B on chromosome 13 causes it.

The build-up of copper in the cornea causes Kayser–Fleischer rings – a brownish pigmentation. Wilson's disease leads to anaemia, kidney and heart problems, pancreatitis, menstrual disorders, miscarriages and premature osteoporosis.

78. D They show a tendency to appear in the later stages of the disease.

Unfortunately, the neuropsychiatric features of SLE are quite varied and lack any particular form or pattern. Mental disorders are the most common neuropsychiatric manifestations. Most of them are usually transient and clear up within 6 weeks and rarely within 6 months. However, they are recurrent and tend to develop when other systemic features relapse. Headache is perhaps the most common symptom of neurological manifestations, often with migraine features. Other neuropsychiatric manifestations include cognitive impairment, mood and anxiety disorders, psychosis, seizures, polyneuropathy and cerebrovascular disease.

79. E Paranoid features figure prominently in psychosis.

The psychosis in myxoedema shows features of delirium, florid delusions and hallucinations. Auditory hallucinations are particularly common. There is a profound loss of interest; mental sluggishness and mood change indicate apathy rather than depression. The memory is affected from the early stages and person is forgetful of day-to-day things. Myxoedema may present with prominent paranoid features. Depressive psychosis does not respond readily to treatment by psychotropic medications until myxoedema has been treated successfully.

80. A Depression is the most common psychiatric presentation in Cushing's syndrome due to pituitary involvement.

However, this is not the case in Cushing's syndrome caused by direct adrenal involvement, e.g. adrenal adenoma or carcinoma. Psychiatric disturbances are found in more than 50% of patients. Severe psychosis often presents with accompanying depression, paranoia and auditory hallucinations with marked fluctuations. Physical changes include moon face, buffalo hump and purple striae on the abdomen with early weight gain. A plethoric complexion with hirsutism, excessive bruising, skin pigmentation and hypertension occurs with mild glycosuria.

81. B It follows a more severe course when the onset is early.

In Huntington's disease (HD), the ratio of incidence in males and females is equal. It rarely skips a generation in its presentation. Choreoathetoid movements usually start in the face, hands and shoulders, and may lead to a dance-like ataxia. Hemichorea may also be seen. Some patients develop striate rigidity rather than chorea, especially when the onset is at an early age. This variant is called the 'Westphal variant' which is associated with tremor, akinesia and cogwheel rigidity, and at times progresses to torsion dystonia. Fits are more common in this variant (16% compared with 3% in general HD). Dementia follows involuntary movements. Recall is particularly impaired, and slowing of cognition is generally marked from the start. Rigid thinking with an inability to change from one subject to another is impaired. It follows a more severe course when the onset is early. Dysarthria often presents early in the disease. The abnormal movements cease during sleep. Psychiatric changes usually occur years before the diagnosis is fully established. There is a change of disposition, emotional lability and paranoia. Depression is usually severe with a high risk of suicide in the early stages (accounts for 7% deaths in non-hospitalised patients). It usually responds to medication or ECT. If psychosis occurs first, delusions are usually followed by hallucinations (delusional–hallucinatory).

82. B Life events are common in the 6 months before an act of parasuicide.

Parasuicide has been defined by Norman Kreitman as any act deliberately undertaken by a person who mimics the act of suicide, but that does not result in a fatal outcome. It is a self-initiated and deliberate act in which the person injures him- or herself, or takes a substance in a quantity that exceeds the therapeutic dose (if any) or his or her habitual level of consumption, and that he or she believes to be pharmacologically active. Most cases of parasuicide are associated with a psychiatric disorder, the most common being: depressive episode, dysthymia, alcohol dependence, personality disorder, etc.

Life events are more common in the 6 months before an act of parasuicide, including:

- Break-up of a relationship
- Being in trouble with the law
- Physical illness
- Illness of a loved one
- Predisposing factors include:
- Marital difficulties
- Unemployment
- Physical illness
- Mental impairment
- Death of one's parent at a young age
- Parental neglect.

83. D Studies of college students have suggested that a quarter meet DSM-IV criteria for BDD.

This is a type of somatoform disorder in which there is a disturbance of body image, and preoccupation with an imagined or slight abnormality in appearance. The person's concern is grossly excessive for a slight physical anomaly. The belief is not of delusional intensity although in clinical practice this distinction is often difficult. Anorexia nervosa fulfils the diagnostic criteria for BDD. The most common age of onset is from adolescence through to the third decade. In psychodynamic theory, BDD has been considered to represent an unconscious displacement on to body parts of sexual or emotional conflicts, feelings of inferiority, poor self-image or guilt. Its co-morbidity includes depression, social anxiety disorder, obsessive–compulsive disorder, agoraphobia, avoidant personality disorder, borderline personality disorder and dependent personality disorder.

84. A About a quarter of new consultations in secondary care will be for medically unexplained symptoms.

This means that doctors treating patients with these symptoms have not found a medical cause, but this does not mean that a medical cause does not exist. These symptoms may be considered synonymous with somatisation disorder. Psychiatric co-morbidity is common in these patients, but the symptoms may not entirely be explained by psychiatric factors. In any week, 60–80% of healthy people experience bodily symptoms, but only a small portion of these will see their GP. About one in five new consultations in primary care will have medically unexplained symptoms. Up to 40% of patients seen by hospital medical specialists have medically unexplained physical symptoms and receive no organic diagnosis.

85. E 40–65%

The percentage risk of developing schizophrenia depends on the relationship to the person with schizophrenia:

- Identical monozygotic twins: 40–65%
- Fraternal twins: 0–15%
- Children of both parents with schizophrenia: 40%
- Children: 13%
- Parents: 6%
- First cousin: 2%.

86. E Urinary incontinence can occur in this condition.

Pseudo-seizures are paroxysmal episodes that resemble epileptic seizures. They are often misdiagnosed as epileptic seizures. Of patients with refractory seizures, 20–30% are considered to have pseudo-seizures. About a third (10–30%) of patients with pseudo-seizures have coexisting epilepsy. It is difficult to differentiate between true seizures and pseudo-seizures by clinical observation alone. During the episode of a pseudo-seizure, patients can present with tongue bite, urinary incontinence or falls, which are generally absent. In the post-ictal phase, the gag and papillary reflexes are retained and there is an increase in prolactin levels. Pseudo-seizures are psychological in origin but can be organic, e.g. syncope, migraine and transient ischaemic attacks. The most conclusive test for differentiating pseudo-seizures from epilepsy is long-term video-EEG recording. Psychiatric disorders that resemble pseudo-seizures include factitious disorder, malingering, panic disorder, schizophrenia and depersonalisation disorder.

87. A Hyperreligiosity

The Gastaut–Geschwind syndrome is associated with involvement of temporolimbic lobe and temporal lobe epilepsy. It can present with some behavioural problems such as hyperreligiosity, exaggerated philosophical concern, hypergraphia, hyposexuality, circumstantiality, intense mental life, or interpersonal 'stickiness' or viscosity. It can also present with increased violence and hostility in the interictal period.

88. A Better response to antipsychotics

Late-onset schizophrenia is characterised by more positive symptoms, fewer negative symptoms and less affective blunting. Patients have a less formal thought disorder, better neuropsychological functioning and better response to antipsychotics. Many of these patients need low-dose antipsychotics to have good symptom control.

89. D Recurrent depression

A literature review demonstrated the strong link of depression with cardiovascular disease. This was observed in patients of all age groups.

90. D Increasing age

Seizure threshold is affected by many factors. It increases with age and is higher in men than in women. Seizure threshold is decreased by most antidepressants and antipsychotics, whereas benzodiazepines and anticonvulsants increase it. Seizure threshold increases during the course of ECT but returns to baseline within a few months of stopping it.

91. C Parents with a forensic history

There are several wide-ranging factors associated with development of conduct disorders in children. **Table 1.3** describes some of the common associations.

Table 1.3 Factors associated with conduct disorders in children

Association	Disorders
Inner city, isolated communities	Increased risk of all child psychiatric disorders
Low maternal education	Externalising disorders, separation disorder
Parental sociopathy	Conduct disorder and oppositional defiant disorder
Family dysfunction	Conduct disorder, hyperactivity, emotional disorders
Mothers with internalising disorders	Children with externalising disorders, e.g. ADHD

92. B Figures of overall prevalence are similar across cultures around the world.

The community prevalence of psychiatric disorders is 2–30%. This reduces to 12–15% when only moderate-to-severe diagnoses are considered. The proportion of girls with psychiatric diagnoses relative to boys increases with age, but overall prevalence is higher for boys. The figures for overall prevalence of childhood and adolescent mental disorders are similar across cultures around the world.

93. A Childhood depression is associated with higher rates of depression in adult life.

The point prevalence of major depression and dysthymia in children is 2%, and 2–5% for adolescents. Depression is equally common in boys and girls up to adolescence. There is a high rate of recovery but a high rate of relapse in children with depressive illness. Childhood or adolescent depression is associated with higher rates of depression in adult life.

94. D Teaching begins at the clinic and then is gradually taken home.

This was developed by Eyberg at the University of Florida. The therapy is delivered to teach parents to build a warm relationship with the child and to teach the child how to behave appropriately. The aim of the therapy is to improve the quality of child–parent relationships, and consists of two phases. The therapist sits behind a one-way mirror and guides the parents with a microphone.

95. E Risperidone

Antipsychotic drugs are the most widely studied drugs in autistic spectrum disorders. They act by dopamine receptor blockade and help to reduce maladaptive behaviours such as stereotypies and self-harm. Selected medications for use in domains of behaviours in autism include:

- Stereotypical and compulsive/repetitive behaviours: SSRIs (fluoxetine/fluvoxamine) and atypical antipsychotics (risperidone)
- Irritability, aggression and self-injury: atypical antipsychotics (risperidone), opiate antagonist (naltrexone) and typical antipsychotics (haloperidol)
- Hyperkinesia and inattention: methylphenidate, α_2-receptor agonist (clonidine) and atomoxetine
- Depressive symptoms: SSRIs
- Manic symptoms: anticonvulsant mood stabiliser (valproate/divalproex)
- Anxiety symptoms: SSRIs and buspirone
- Sleep dysfunction: melatonin and an antihistamine

96. B Family therapy

NICE guidelines on depression give guidance on the management of depression based on its severity. Mild and moderate depressive episodes are mainly treated (first line) with psychological therapies, i.e. cognitive–behavioural therapy (CBT), interpersonal therapy or family therapy. In severe depressive episodes, medication is the first-line treatment. However, we should be careful in choosing therapy for children and adolescents.

97. A 13%

There was a report that 13.2% of the young people questioned in a trial had tried to harm themselves at some point in their lives, 6.9% in the previous year; 15% had reported thoughts of suicide and 54% of those reporting self-harm described more than one episode/incident. The presentation to hospital was described in only 12.6% of adolescents who had engaged in self-harm.

98. D Separation anxiety

School refusal can be the presenting complaint for children with a variety of underlying disorders, with separation anxiety being the most common diagnosis, particularly among younger children. In many cases, school refusal results from the combination of a child who does not want to separate and parents who do not insist on school attendance. This is because either they have difficulty imposing limits in general or they share their child's anxieties about separation.

99. A Citalopram

Treatment of severe depression in children presents a challenge because there are limited options available compared with the adult population. NICE guidelines provide useful information to meet this challenge (Table 1.4).

Table 1.4 Pharmacological treatment for depression in children and adolescents: UK and US guidelines and licensing of antidepressants

Drug	NICE	Texas[a]	UK	USA
Citalopram	Second line	First line	18+	18+
Escitalopram	Not discussed	Second line	18+	12+
Fluoxetine	First line	First line	8+[b]	8+
Paroxetine	Contraindicated by the CSM	Second line[c]	18+	18+
Sertraline	Second line	First line	18+	18+
Venlafaxine	Contraindicated by the CSM	Third line	18+	18+

CSM, Committee on Safety of Medicines; NICE, National Institute for Health and Care Excellence; Texas, Texas Children's Medication Algorithm Project.
[a] For major depression of sufficient severity to warrant medication.
[b] For moderate-to-severe depression.
[c] Adolescents only.

100. E About 10% of autistic individuals go through a phase in adolescence when they lose language skills.

Autistic individuals are not at an increased risk of developing schizophrenia in adult life. Even with IQ and speech on their side, autistic children have only around a 50% chance of a good social outcome in adult life. Autistic aloofness tends to improve with time in just over half of all cases. Autistic children who do not have useful speech by age 5 rarely go on to develop it. Sometimes, there is intellectual deterioration as well. The decline is not progressive, but the lost skills are not generally regained.

101. B Conduct disorder

Most psychological traits have been found to have a heritability of around 40–60%. This means that genetic differences between individuals account for roughly half the observed variance in a given population. Conduct problems are the one probable exception to this rule, with most (but not all) studies showing a small genetic contribution. Conduct disorders commonly cluster in families but, compared with other child psychiatric disorders, shared environment has a proportionally greater influence than shared genes. Although twin studies have shown high concordance for monozygotic pairs, the concordance for dizygotic pairs is also high. Adoption studies have shown the influence of biological parents to be less than that of the adoptive ones. However, they show a strong interactive effect whereby a difficult temperament (indexed by antisocial behaviour in biological parents) and unfavourable environment (as indexed by antisocial behaviour in the adoptive parents) leads to a far higher rate of antisocial behaviour and criminality than would be expected by addition.

102. E Parent management training

This is the best-established approach for managing conduct disorders, with numerous randomised controlled trials attesting to its effectiveness. It gets parents to pay attention to desired behaviour; positive aspects of child–parent relationships are promoted and parents are taught effective techniques for handling undesirable behaviour. It can be given more economically in groups while maintaining effectiveness.

103. A Down's syndrome

This is due to full trisomy 21 (47,XX +21 or 47,XY + 21) in 95% of people. Robertsonian translocation between acrocentric chromosomes accounts for another 5%. The trisomy occurs from anew. Shuttleworth made two interesting observations in 1909: Down's syndrome children tended to be the youngest of their siblings and Down's syndrome was associated with advanced maternal age. Non-disjunction is the common mechanism. Down's syndrome is the most common example of a genetic condition that is not inherited. It occurs in 1:600–1:1000 newborns.

104. A Men with Down's syndrome due to non-disjunction have a high incidence of infertility.

The development of sexuality is an issue for patients with Down's syndrome. Down's syndrome girls start menstruating at almost the same age as other girls and have ovulatory cycles. Women with Down's syndrome are known to have had children. However, the fertility rate is significantly lower than in the general population, probably due to slow follicular development in the ovaries, and complete failure to ovulate in some women. Menopause occurs on average 5 years early in these women. Most of the men have reduced sperm counts due to unknown causes. Men with mosaic Down's syndrome are fertile and have been known to have children. However, men with full trisomy 21 are usually infertile.

Answers: MCQs

105. B 20–40%

The prevalence of psychiatric morbidity is 4–10 times that in the general population. Overall, 20–40% have a concurrent psychiatric illness excluding behavioural problems. Proposed reasons for this include:

- Higher rates in families with a genetic predisposition
- Higher prevalence of learning disability and mental illness in lower socioeconomic groups
- Vulnerable population
- Increased exposure to abuse
- Multiple traumatic life experiences
- Lack of early ego-strengthening experiences (e.g. lack of consistent primary caregiver)
- Lack of protective life experiences, e.g. employment, close confiding relationships
- Neurochemical abnormalities associated with organic brain abnormalities
- Increased rates of other risk factors for mental illness, e.g. epilepsy, sensory impairments
- Syndrome-specific psychiatric risk associated with genetic phenotype, e.g. obsessive–compulsive disorder is associated with Down's syndrome.

106. A Age-specific prevalence varies over time.

The point prevalence of severe intellectual impairment varies between similar cohorts (concurrent age groups) in different communities, e.g. 1.62/1000 children born in 1951–55 in Salford, England, and 7.34/1000 born in 1957 in Amsterdam, The Netherlands. A greater variation is expected in developing countries. Age-specific prevalence varies over time in the same community. A similar pattern of temporal variation is common throughout the developed world, e.g. increases have been the result of decreased early mortality and increased survival associated with better neonatal care. More recently, amniocentesis and abortion programmes have reduced Down's syndrome prevalence. Prevalence varies by age because of cohort differences from birth and early infancy. Prevalence varies by age and time because survival has increased at all ages. There are usually more men than women at all ages. Studies have tended to show a social class gradient consistent with the known social distribution of morbidity and mortality.

107. B Handicap

Impairment is the loss or abnormality of structure or function. Disability means the restriction or lack of ability to perform an activity in the manner or within the range considered normal for a person. Handicap means the disadvantage for an individual that prevents or limits his or her usual performance or role (**Table 1.5**)

Table 1.5 Assessment of impairment, disability and handicap	
Impairment	Established tests of intellectual functioning, e.g. the Wechsler scales
Disability	Established assessments of functioning, e.g. Vineland Adaptive Behaviour Scales, American Adaptive Behaviour Scales, Hampshire Assessment for Living with Others (HALO)
Handicap	Assessments of quality of life and life experiences, e.g. Life Experiences Checklist

108. D Offences are broadly similar to those of offenders without learning disability.

Offending in learning disability is:

- More likely in mild and moderate than in severe learning disability
- More likely in association with family, social and environmental disadvantage.

Offences are broadly similar to those of offenders without learning disability. There is some evidence that there are increased rates of sex offending and fire-raising in LD individuals.

Learning disability together with antisocial personality features carries a high risk for offending. There has been a recent fall in the use of compulsory admission for people with a learning disability.

Property offences are often committed with a lack of forethought and are opportunistic. People with learning disability are more commonly victims of crime and many of them do not report them to the police. These people put themselves at risk, perhaps due to lack of understanding of social norms and conventions, and chronic low self-esteem. They are more likely to be suggestible at interview and to give false confessions. They are more likely to commit sexual offences, especially against young children and boys. Arson has been consistently associated with learning disability in those referred for hospital treatment.

109. A Family members are more likely to have borderline or mild intellectual disability.

Mild or borderline intellectual impairment is more common in families of lower socioeconomic status. There are no dysmorphic features in the affected person as well as in family members.

110. A Batten's disease

This is also called juvenile neuronal ceroid lipofuscinosis (NCL) and Spielmeyer–Vogt–Sjögren–Batten disease. It is an autosomal recessive neurodegenerative disease. It is very rare (2–4 in 100 000 births) but life threatening. Parry's disease is the adult form of NCL. The earlier the onset of illness, the poorer the prognosis. Early symptoms (visual difficulties, seizures) usually appear around the age of 2–10 years. The muscles have abnormally high tone (myoclonus) with a lack of coordination. There can be dementia or mental impairment with a compromised mental ability. The patients may present with movement disorders such as choreoathetosis, unsteady gait (ataxia) or seizures.

111. D Single word reading

The primary skill deficit in dyslexia is difficulty at the level of single word reading. The word-reading problems arise from core cognitive deficits in phonological processing which consist of:

- Poor phonological awareness of the phonological structure of words in one's language
- Difficulties in mastering the alphabetic principle, i.e. connecting written letters (graphemes) with speech sounds (phonemes).

Other prominent impairments seen in most if not all people with dyslexia are poor phonological working memory and impaired rapid autonomic naming. Higher linguistic skills such as syntactic and semantic processing skills are largely intact.

112. C PCL-R (Hare)

Actuarial tools attach specific statistical weighting to different variables to assess the risk. The common example in day-to-day life is car insurance quotations, which are compiled using actuarial tools. Other examples include: the Violence Risk Appraisal Guide (VRAG) which is a 12-item actuarial tool for violence risk assessment and includes the PCL-R as a subscale; Violence risk scale; the Static-99; and the SORAG (Sexual Risk Offender Appraisal Guide).

In contrast, structured professional judgement guides consider a number of variables, which will have some application to the assessment of risk in the case under consideration. This allows more flexibility to account for case-specific influences and context, and moves the emphasis from prediction to risk management.

This question asks for violence risk assessment tools. It does not specify what form of violence, so the candidate must assume that it means physical and sexual violence. Therefore, the ESR-20 should be immediately eliminated, because this is the Estimate of Suicide Risk and a structured professional judgement tool. All the possible answers except the PCL-R (Psychopathy Checklist revised) are structured professional judgement risk assessment tools. The Historical, Clinical, Risk Management-20 (HCR-20) is a well-known tool for formulating violence risk that is commonly used within forensic settings. The Risk for Sexual Violence Protocol (RSVP) and Sexual Violence Risk-20 (SVR-20) are specific to sexual violence.

113. B *Actus reus*

In all offences, it must be proven beyond reasonable doubt that the accused physically did the act, which is known as *actus reus*. In most offences, it must also be proven that the defendant's intention or attitude of mind was as required for the crime in question (known as having the necessary *mens rea*). Therefore, for a crime to be committed the accused should have done the act but must also have intent. Children under the age of 10 in England and Wales, and 8 in Scotland are assumed to be incapable of forming criminal intent.

114. A 4%

There has been a review of 62 surveys from prisons in 12 countries; 3.7% of the men had psychotic illnesses. This compares with a figure from the Office for National Statistics (ONS) for the community sample of 0.4%. Prisoners were several times more likely (almost 20 times) to have psychosis and major depression (10–12%) and approximately 10 times more likely to have antisocial personality disorder than the general population. Antisocial personality disorder was exhibited in 47% of male and 21% of female prisoners. Female prisoners show a higher rate of neurotic disorders, substance misuse and self-harm than men. Treatment in the absence of a prisoner's informed consent is not permitted. However, treatment for mental disorders is permitted under mental health legislation.

115. B 1%

Homicide–suicide describes the situation when a person kills someone (often a spouse or relative) and then takes his or her own life. In England and Wales, it is estimated that homicide–suicide accounts for 1% of all homicides. It has been found that a firearm was the most frequently used method for the homicide and suicide, and approximately one in four perpetrators failed in the suicide attempt.

116. E Stages 3–4

Offending can occur during sleep, in which case a defence of automatism is appropriate. Sleepwalking occurs during stages 3–4 of slow-wave sleep, not REM sleep when the body is normally paralysed.

It has been suggested that the following factors are necessary for the diagnosis of sleepwalking, especially in relation to assessment of individuals charged under the criminal justice system. The general factors are:

- Family history: there is a known genetic element to the aetiology of sleepwalking.
- Childhood onset: sleepwalking commonly begins in childhood, with a lower proportion starting during adolescence.
- Late-onset of sleepwalking is rare, and more likely after a head injury. Be suspicious if sleepwalking occurs for the first time at the time of the offence.

Specific factors include:

- Sleepwalking occurs in stages 3–4 of sleep and should therefore occur within 2 hours of going to sleep.
- The person should be disoriented on awakening.
- Any witnesses should report inappropriate automatic behaviours and disorientation on awakening.
- There should be amnesia for the whole period of sleepwalking.
- Trigger factors may be present, including drugs, alcohol, excessive fatigue and stress.
- If the crime is a sexual one, sexual arousal during sleep occurs only during REM sleep and would therefore not occur during sleepwalking.
- Any memories from before the sleepwalking should be non-narrative and non-dream like.
- It is unusual for there to be any attempt to conceal a crime committed during sleepwalking.
- There may have been similar behaviours during previous sleepwalking episode.
- If the crime appears to be motiveless and out of character, this would give some support to it being committed during sleepwalking.

117. B Arson

There is growing evidence that people with Asperger's syndrome are more likely to commit fire-setting offences than people without the syndrome. Both alcohol and drug misuse and drug offences have been reported in this population, although substance misuse is comparatively rare. Epidemiological studies indicate that people with Asperger's syndrome do commit sexual offences, but there is evidence that the rates of sexual offending in general, and of child sex offences in particular, are lower among offenders with autistic spectrum disorders.

118. B Being unfit to plead can result in a trial of facts.

Fitness to plead is concerned with a defendant's mental state at the time of trial. The principle of being unfit to plead, which is also known as being under disability, was first established in statute in section 2 of the Criminal Lunatics Act 1800. The tests of disability are derived from the case of a deaf mute (*R v Pritchard 1836*) and the judgment is interpreted today as follows: to be considered fit to plead, the defendant must have the capacity to:

- understand the charge
- instruct a lawyer
- challenge a juror
- plead to the charge
- understand the evidence.

A trial of facts is where a jury, hearing evidence, determines whether the accused 'did the act or made the omission against him'. It is important to understand that this does not amount to a finding of guilt. If not satisfied on this issue, the jury return a verdict of acquittal.

119. A It can be caused by an insulinoma.

This question addresses the candidate's knowledge of automatism. Automatism is a rare plea in which the defendant claims, at the time of the offence, that he was behaving 'automatically' and therefore is not guilty of a crime. The legal definition (*Bratty v AG for Northern Ireland* 1963) defines automatism, as 'the state of a person who, though capable of action, is not conscious of what he is doing'. It means an unconscious involuntary action and it is therefore a defence because the mind does not go with what is being done. It is argued that in automatism there is no conscious capacity to control one's actions and therefore no possibility of *mens rea*.

There are two forms of automatism:

1. Sane automatism: due to external causes (one-off) such as concussion after a blow to the head or a confusional state after an anaesthetic. Hypoglycaemia after a large insulin injection would also apply. A successful plea of sane automatism results in complete acquittal of the charge.

2. Insane automatism: due to internal causes of behaviour without voluntary control. Examples include epilepsy, insulinoma (causing episodes of hypoglycaemia) and degenerative brain diseases. A successful plea of insane automatism would lead to the defendant being found not guilty by reason of insanity and therefore the McNaughton rules apply.

120. D Polyneuropathy and cirrhosis of the liver

EM Jellinek (1890–1963) was a biostatistician, physiologist and prominent researcher in alcoholism. He developed classification of alcoholism as follows:

- α alcoholism: this is the earliest stage of alcoholism characterised by psychological dependence on alcohol to relieve physical or psychological pain. He called them 'problem drinkers' because their drinking causes personal and social problems. These people can stop drinking if they are determined to do so because they have not lost control and do not have a 'disease'.
- β alcoholism: people with this problem drink alcohol heavily, but do not have physical addiction or withdrawal symptoms or a 'disease'. They do, however, have polyneuropathy and/or cirrhosis of the liver.
- γ alcoholism: people with this problem have developed tissue tolerance and physical dependence. They have lost control over their drinking and have a 'disease'.
- δ alcoholism: they have features of γ alcoholism with an inability to abstain minus loss of control.
- ϵ alcoholism: this is a fully fledged disease, which manifests as dipsomania or periodic alcoholism.

121. D Three or more manifestations must be present for more than a month.

Three or more manifestations should have occurred together for at least 1 month or occurred together repeatedly within a 12-month period. Tolerance refers to diminished effects with use of the same amount of intake of the substance. A strong desire to take the substance is one of the manifestations that may be present. A physiological withdrawal state should be evident when substance use is stopped or reduced. Continuing to take a substance with clear evidence of harm is one of the manifestations of a dependence syndrome.

122. E Partial remission

In patients with alcohol or substance dependence, additional code specifiers may be used to describe the condition further. These code specifiers help us to understand further whether the person is currently abstinent; if so is he in a protective environment such as a rehab setting or is he on treatment? On the other hand, if he is still dependent, this describes the pattern of substance dependence.

123. A Cognitive–behavioural therapy

Psychological interventions, such as CBT, behavioural therapies or social network- and environment-based therapies, should be offered to people with harmful drinking and mild alcohol dependence. Such therapies should also be offered after successful withdrawal from moderate-to-severe alcohol dependence. Family therapy should be considered in children and adolescents who misuse alcohol.

124. A GABA agonism

Although the exact mechanism is not known, acamprosate is thought to activate GABA (γ-aminobutyric acid) receptors and block glutamatergic NMDA (N-methyl-D-aspartate) receptors. The mechanism of action involves functional antagonism of ionotropic NMDA receptors. It is noted that direct reactions between acamprosate and NMDA receptors are weak. It is also suggested that there are other possible mechanisms of action. Acamprosate may modulate NMDA receptors via regulatory polyamine sites or directly act on metabotropic glutamate receptors.

125. E Specialised cognitive–behavioural therapy

The leading treatment for bulimia nervosa is a specific form of CBT. There is strong research evidence for this treatment and it is recommended in the NICE guidance. Interpersonal psychotherapy offers an evidence-based alternative to CBT and involves about the same amount of therapist contact. However, interpersonal psychotherapy has considerably less empirical support than CBT and takes longer to achieve comparable effects. However, NICE recommends that it should be considered as an alternative to CBT. Both antidepressant drugs and certain self-help programmes have some efficacy and are relatively straightforward to implement. However, as the evidence suggests that a few patients make a full and long-lasting response to either treatment, NICE recommends that these treatments be viewed as possible first steps in management. Fluoxetine 60 mg/day is the antidepressant of choice.

126. A It occurs in organic pathological states.

Capgras' syndrome is a delusional misidentification. The patient believes that an imposter pretending to be that person has replaced someone close to him or her; the abnormality is delusional, not hallucinatory. It is a rare occurrence, which may form part of a schizophrenic illness or affective disorder. Uncommonly it may occur in organic states. In Capgras' syndrome, there is no outward change in the appearance of the objects and there is no false perception because the patient admits that the double exactly resembles the original.

127. A It is a common motivation for homicide.

Morbid jealousy is a disorder of thought content and it may take various forms, e.g. as a delusion, overvalued idea, depressive affect or anxiety state. It is also known as Othello's syndrome. It occurs in men more often than women. It may be present on its own or as a symptom of schizophrenia, alcohol abuse or cocaine abuse. It is a common cause of domestic abuse and is associated with homicide. The risk of harm is more towards the partner than the rival person alleged to be in the relationship.

128. B Hyperaesthesia

Increased intensity of sensations (hyperaesthesia) may be the result of intense emotions or a lowering of the physiological threshold. Examples include seeing roof tiles as brilliant flaming red or hearing the noise of a door closing like a clap of thunder. Anxiety and depressive disorders, as well as hangovers from alcohol and migraine, are all associated with increased sensitivity to noise (hyperacusis). Dysmegalopsia refers to changes in the perceived shapes of objects. There are two types: micropsia, which refers to seeing objects smaller than their actual size, and macropsia, which refers to seeing objects larger than they actually are. Dysmegalopsia results from retinal disease, accommodation and convergence problems, and temporal and parietal lobe lesions. An illusion refers to misrepresentations of stimuli arising from external objects. There are three types of illusions: complete illusions, affect illusions and pareidolia.

129. C Couvade's syndrome

This is an abnormality of self-experience when a man also complains of obstetric symptoms during his partner's pregnancy and parturition. Gross forms of Couvade's syndrome are very rare, but minor symptoms in the man directly associated with his partner's pregnancy are quite common. Symptoms of Couvade's syndrome in the man occur from the third month of pregnancy onwards (more frequent in months 3 and 9). The symptoms include loss of appetite, toothache, nausea and vomiting (often morning sickness), indigestion, vague abdominal pains, constipation and diarrhoea. Anxiety, tension, insomnia and emotional instability are common complaints and there is a preoccupation with his partner's condition. The chronological relationship with the partner's pregnancy is more important for making the diagnosis than the nature of the symptoms. It is not delusional. The man with Couvade's syndrome does not believe himself to be pregnant. Cotard's syndrome refers to a condition in which people believe that they are dead or have nihilistic delusions. Autoscopy is also known as phantom mirror image. It is the experience of seeing oneself and recognising that it is oneself. It can occur in healthy people when they are tired or emotionally exhausted. Autoscopy can also occur in patients with schizophrenia and organic brain disorders.

130. A Cognitive–analytic therapy

- Factors favouring integrative, structured brief therapy (e.g. cognitive–analytic therapy or CAT): when the issues are more complex and intertwined and related to particular stressors, typically definable pattern of relationship issues, and ongoing and repeated self-limiting but avoided themes.
- Factors favouring short-term dynamic therapy: when the problems are clear and definable, and conflicts are more focal than general. The aim of the therapy is to achieve limited goals in a limited time and the problems are more 'oedipal' in nature, e.g. competition anxiety, authority and power problems, conflict in triangular relationships and anxiety in sexual relationships. There should be enough trust between the patient and the therapist to help in tolerating the frustration that might surface during the therapy.
- Factors favouring CBT: abnormal thought patterns (cognition) or behaviours that are maintaining dysfunctional patterns in the person's life. The patient is aware of the problem and doesn't have any overwhelming relationship issues that may interfere in establishing a therapeutic relationship.
- Factors for long-term individual therapy: there is a lack of clarity about the problems, the conflicts are not clearly definable, there are severe difficult personality issues, and the goals of the therapy can be defined in terms of general interpersonal function, i.e. control or intimacy.

Answers: EMIs

131. A Correlation coefficient
This indicates the degree to which two measures are related although it does not explain how.

132. B Kendall's correlational coefficient
This is a correlational coefficient for two categorical or non-parametrically (non-normally) distributed variables.

133. C Logistic regression
This is used when the dependent variable is of a dichotomous or binary type (e.g. yes or no) whereas the independent variable can be of any type.

134. D Multiple analysis of co-variance
This is used with multiple dependent and independent variables.

135. E Multiple analysis of variance
This is used with multiple dependent variables.

136. B Blinding
This means that both the participants and the investigators are unaware of the information about which group the participants are allocated to. This is to avoid any bias that could arise in the study.

137. E Recall bias
When compared with healthy control participants, individuals with the disorder are likely to have increased health awareness and greater understanding of the disease process. 'Response priming' can occur in a study with participants who have chronic conditions. The ability to recall past events accurately varies from person to person. This is a problem in retrospective studies. Multiple sources of information help corroborate data.

138. C Matching
In this scenario, controlled participants are selected based on certain characteristics (usually potential confounding factors) that they have in common with experimental participants. This is done to ensure that confounders are distributed in both groups.

139. F Restriction

This is a way of achieving reduction of confounding factors. In this study, they were focusing on non-cannabis-related factors in schizophrenia.

140. G Stratification

In this study, economics status was a confounding factor, hence the data stratification.

141. J Synaesthesia

The word 'synaesthesia' originated from 'syn', a Greek word meaning together and 'aesthesia' meaning sensation. Psychomimetic drugs such as LSD can induce multiple perceptual changes at the same time, including changes in spatial orientation, perception of movement, colour appreciation, visual illusions and hallucinations at once. Synaesthesia occurs when a stimulus image in one sensory modality is perceived as an image in another sensory modality. It is not an image in the mind's eye; the experience is real and is projected outside the individual. He can describe the colour, shape and taste of someone's voice.

142. B Charles Bonnet syndrome

This is a syndrome (phantom visual images) in which the patient experiences complex visual hallucinations that are not associated with any other psychiatric abnormality. It usually occurs with loss of vision. Although more common in elderly people, it can occur at any age and follows central or peripheral vision loss. It can last from days to years and patient can see human images, animals, buildings, and static or moving scenery.

143. K Temporal lobe epilepsy (TLE)

Auditory and visual hallucinations can occur synchronously in pathological organic states of TLE.

Children with complex febrile seizures lasting >15 min have focal features, or recur within 24 hours. Relationship of TLE with childhood febrile convulsions is controversial. Other causes of TLE include head trauma resulting in encephalomalacia or cortical scarring, infections such as meningitis, vascular malformations such as arteriovenous malformations, traumatic delivery such as forceps deliveries, hamartomas in the brain, meningiomas, etc., cryptogenic (of obscure origin) and rarely idiopathic (genetic).

144. D Delirium tremens

This is an acute organic condition due to alcohol withdrawal, coloured by gross changes in perception mood and conscious state. The perceptual disturbance usually starts with pareidolic or affective illusions followed by visual and the haptic lilliputian hallucinations. These experiences are in a constant state of flux rapidly changing from one form to the other, causing confusion and terror in the patients. Illusions are usually mixed with hallucinations and are very frightening. There is a high level of suggestibility in patients at these times, which can lead to abnormal visual experience as a result of suggestibility.

145. B CATIE

Thus is an acronym for 'Clinical Antipsychotic Trials of Intervention Effectiveness'. It assessed the effectiveness of antipsychotic medication used in the treatment of schizophrenia and compared older antipsychotics with newer antipsychotics. The antipsychotics used in the trial were perphenazine (first generation) and second-generation drugs: olanzapine, quetiapine, risperidone and ziprasidone. It was a double-blind randomized trial. The follow-up period was for 18 months. The primary measure was to check the duration for which a patient remained on medication.

146. I SOHO

Schizophrenia Outpatient Health Outcomes study (SOHO) is an observational study of outpatients who received antipsychotic medication for the treatment of schizophrenia. Ten European countries participated in the study. Data on more than 9000 patients was analysed in the study.

147. D DEPRES

This was the first pan-European survey of depression in the community in 1990. In the second phase of the study six depressed patient types were identified with clearly differentiated profiles based on cluster analysis of the data. It was set up to examine depression across six European countries including the UK. The most commonly experienced symptoms of depression were low mood (76%), tiredness (73%) and sleep problems (63%). SmithKline Beecham Pharmaceuticals funded the study. The study demonstrated that 17% of the general population has depression. More patients on SSRIs felt like normal self than those on tricyclic antidepressants.

148. E ESEMeD

This was conducted in six studies across Europe, namely Belgium, France, Germany, Italy, the Netherlands and Spain. It was initially named the European Study of the Epidemiology of Mental Disorders/Mental Health Disability (ESEMeD/MHEDEA). The age range of participants was ≥18 years. It was a cross-sectional study. Patients receiving medication and/or psychological therapies were considered in the study. Assessments took place in the community with the help of computer-assisted techniques. Questionnaires were based on CIDI (Composite International Diagnostic Interview).

149. H POTS

This was conducted in three academic centres across the USA. It was conducted to evaluate the efficacy of CBT alone, sertraline alone, and CBT and sertraline combined. The duration of treatment was 12 weeks and participants were recruited between September 1997 and December 2002. The findings of the study suggested that children and adolescents should begin treatment with either a combination of CBT and a SSRI or CBT alone.

150. C CUtLASS 1

This study essentially compared first-generation antipsychotics with second-generation antipsychotics (except clozapine) in the treatment of schizophrenia. The outcome measure used was quality of life. The results showed no significant improvement in the outcome in any of the groups. Interestingly patients on first-generation antipsychotics showed better quality of life compared with second-generation antipsychotics **Table 1.6**

Table 1.6 Abbreviations of studies

AESOP	Aetiology and Ethnicity of Schizophrenia and Other Psychoses
CAFÉ	Comparison of Atypicals in First Episode of psychosis
CATIE	Clinical Antipsychotic Trials of Intervention Effectiveness
CUtLASS	Cost Utility of the Latest Antipsychotic Drugs in Schizophrenia Study
DEPRES	Depression Research in European Society
DOSMD	Determinants of Outcome of Severe Mental Disorders
ESEMeD	European Study of the Epidemiology of Mental Disorders
EUFEST	European First Episode Schizophrenia Trial
IPSS	International Pilot Study of Schizophrenia
MTA	Multimodal Treatment of ADHD
NEMESIS	Netherlands Mental Health Survey and Incidence Study
POTS	Pediatric OCD Treatment Study
SOHO	Schizophrenia outpatient health outcomes
STAR*D	Sequenced Treatment Alternatives to Relieve Depression (STAR*D)
TADS	Treatment for Adolescents with Depression Study
TEOSS	Treatment of Early Onset Schizophrenia Spectrum disorders
TORDIA	Treatment Of SSRI Resistant Depression in Adolescents

151. D Point prevalence

This refers to the proportion of people affected by the condition or disease in study in a defined population at a specified period of time.

152. A Cumulative incidence

This measures the proportion of people developing a disease or disorder in a specified population over a period of time. Hence, as the time period of study increases, cumulative incidence would also increase. It ranges from 0 to 1. The time period is also mentioned.

153. F Standardised mortality rate

The mortality rate is the incidence rate that expresses the risk of death in a population over a time period. It is often useful to have a single measure of mortality for a given population, which allows for the make-up of that population to compare different populations on one measure rather than several measures. An adjustment or standardisation process achieves this.

Life-time prevalence refers to the proportion of people who had a given condition or disease at least once in their lifetime in a given population.

Morbidity rate refers to the rate measuring the occurrence of disease in a specified population. Morbidity rates include incidence and prevalence rates.

Standardised mortality ratio: ratio of observed mortality rate to the expected mortality rate in the population.

Period prevalence: the proportion of the population that has the disease in a given period.

154. B Play the winner

In this approach, the first participant is allocated by simple randomisation, and thereafter every subsequent allocation is based on the success or failure of the immediate preceding participant.

155. F Randomisation permutated blocks

This requires randomisation in a group of, say, four, six, etc. to ensure that the numbers are equal in the two groups.

156. D Stratified randomisation

This divides the participants into homogeneous subgroups before sampling. The strata should be mutually exclusive, i.e. every element in the population must be assigned to only one stratum/group. It helps to select representative samples by reducing sampling error. It allocates participants on the basis of the same variables, e.g. prognosis, to ensure that they are evenly distributed within the study. However, it requires an additional schedule for each stratum. Stratification can produce a weighted mean that has less variability compared with the arithmetic mean of a random sample.

157. E Randomised consent method

This is used occasionally to lessen the effect of some patients refusing to participate in a study.

158. C Each participant received both the intervention and the treatment, G Separated by a period of no treatment

Cross-over trials are a real option in relatively rare diseases in which the number of available participants may not permit a randomised, parallel-group, controlled trial. The participants act as their own controls. These trials are useful in psychology, education, pharmaceutical science and medicine (diagnosis, treatment and prevention of disease). They offer two advantages over non-crossover studies: the influence of confounding co-variates is reduced and they are statistically efficient because fewer participants are required. They have several disadvantages: historical controls, 'order', 'learning', and 'carry-over' effects. An n-of-1 trial is a special example of a cross-over trial.

159. B Each group receives a different treatment with both groups being entered at the same time, E Results are analysed by comparing groups

Parallel-group comparison is a part of controlled trials that is necessary to evaluate a new treatment against a placebo or gold standard treatment. This comparison sometimes overestimates the therapeutic benefits.

160. D Participants are assessed before and after an intervention, F Results are analysed in terms of differences between participant pairs

In this type of study design, the participants are offered two alternatives and then asked to indicate to the researchers which alternative they like most. Paired comparison can be included in uncontrolled, controlled and randomised controlled trials of new treatments.

Answers: EMIs

161. A Assumes a poor outcome for drop-outs, E Differences in the drop-out rates and the timing of these drop-outs influence the estimation of treatment

Last observation carried forward (LOCF) is an analytical method used to evaluate a missing value in a clinical trial from the last measurement in an individual participant. Participants who drop out for various reasons, such as side effects or ineffective treatment, are considered treatment failures. LOCF may therefore under- or overestimate the benefits of treatment.

162. D Data on all patients entering a trial should be analysed with respect to the groups to which they were originally randomised. regardless of whether or not they received treatment, E Differences in the drop-out rates and the timing of these drop-outs influence the estimation of treatment

Intention-to-treat analysis is a method to analyse the data generated in the course of a clinical trial according to assigned groups. Trial drop-outs are regarded as treatment failures and cannot be ignored in the analysis of data. All clinical trials should conduct intention-to-treat analysis to avoid overestimating the benefits of treatment. Generally, a continuous measure such as a symptom severity score gives more statistical power than a dichotomous or categorical measure. For a continuous measure, LOCF is used as the final measure.

163. C Data should be analysed as unit of randomisation, F Interventions are directed at groups rather than individual participants

Cluster trials are a special type of RCTs in which interventions are directed at groups rather than individuals. They are commonly used in evaluating more global aspects of health services than one particular treatment, or where allocation of participants is not practicable. They require analysis in clusters, i.e. unit of randomisation rather than individuals, which needs a lot of clusters to detect a statistically significant effect.

164. B Investigations, F Staff salaries

Health economics can be applied to various aspects of healthcare such as treatment. They can help to make decisions about value for money by comparing the effects of competing interventions. An economic analysis requires consideration of the underlying research approach and relevant inputs: direct costs (medical expenses), and indirect costs and inputs. Direct costs are the resources consumed by the programme rather than an alternative.

165. C Pain and suffering, E Social stigma

Intangible costs are immeasurable human costs such as pain, suffering stigma, etc.

166. G Value of 'unpaid work', H Work days lost

Indirect costs are productivity gains and losses with the focus on patient time consumed or freed up by healthcare programmes. They are also referred to as overhead costs, e.g. electricity, gas, rental, capital costs.

167. F Health STAR

Health STAR (Health – Services Technology, Administration and Research) contains materials specifically selected with a focus on health services, research and non-clinical aspects of healthcare delivery (e.g. healthcare administration, economics planning and policy).

168. B CINAHL

The Cumulative Index to Nursing and Allied Health Literature (CINAHL) is a database for nursing literature.

169. D EMBASE

This is a database of pharmaceutical and biomedical literature produced by Elsevier. It concentrates on European sources and drug-related literature. The Cochrane Library is a collection of databases, most of which are solely databases of systematic reviews of healthcare interventions. It provides a quick and focused way of locating RCTs. MEDLINE is a major source of published biomedical scientific literature produced by the National Library of Medicine in the USA. It contains thousands of pieces of published data.

170. D Examples include case reports and series, audits, cross-sectional surveys and qualitative study, F Generally conducted without a control group, H Suitable for hypothesis generation

Descriptive studies are generally conducted without a control group, and are suitable only for generating hypotheses. Examples include case reports, case series, audits, cross-sectional surveys of psychiatric morbidity and qualitative studies.

171. C Examples include case–control and cohort studies, E Generally compare two groups, I Suitable for hypothesis testing

Analytical studies include two groups of participants: cases and controls can be healthy participants or those with a different disease. They are suitable for testing a hypothesis. Examples are case–control studies and cohort studies.

172. A Causation can be inferred, B Examples are controlled clinical trial and economic analyses, systematic reviews and their meta-analyses, G Something is given or done in the experimental group but not in the control group

Experimental studies include 'experimental' and control groups. Any resulting differences in outcome are measured, from which causation may be inferred. Examples of experimental studies are controlled clinical trial and economic analyses, systematic reviews and their meta-analysis.

173. G Single blinding

This helps to reduce potential biases. In a single-blind design, the participants are not aware of the treatment that they are receiving, i.e. placebo or active drug.

Answers: EMIs

174. A Double blinding

In a double-blind study design, both the participants and the investigators are not aware of the treatment that the participants are receiving. This design helps to reduce investigators' bias.

175. G Triple blinding

In this design, the analysis of outcome is carried out by independent investigators who are blind to the treatment given. Both the investigators and the participants are unaware of the treatment that the participants are receiving.

176. D Recall bias

This is introduced by selective memory of participants or informants, who are likely to 'search after meaning' and identify possible exposures. It is also sometimes called 'rumination bias', e.g. depressed patients may be more likely to remember adverse life events. Sometimes, participants may alter their responses in the direction that they perceive is desired by the investigators. This is known as 'obsequiousness bias'.

177. B Incidence risk

This is the number of new cases of a disease over a period of time out of the total population at risk. It is also called cumulative incidence because the number developing disease may change over time through death or loss to follow-up.

178. A Incidence density

This is the new cases of a disease out of the total person-time of observation. It is also called the incidence rate. It provides varying person-years of observation, and is more reliable for quantifying the risk of developing a disease over a certain period of time.

179. E Period prevalence

This includes point prevalence (number of new cases in a population at a particular point in time) and new cases over a period of time.

180. G Standardised mortality ratio

This is calculated as the ratio of observed to expected deaths. It can be analysed by parametric or non-parametric statistics depending on their distribution. The mortality rate is an incidence rate that expresses the risk of death in a population over a period of time. It is useful to have a single measure of mortality for a population to allow meaningful comparison between different populations.

181. E Response set

Some individuals have the tendency to either agree or disagree. They may not reveal their true opinion in a research study. It is human nature to alter one's behaviour when we know that we are being observed. This is called attention bias.

182. F Social acceptability

Most people have a tendency to minimise any perceived deviation from the norm, e.g. some relative or the patient minimises the history of substance misuse or other psychiatric symptoms. Some people simply avoid the question altogether, and this is called 'undesirability bias'.

183. D Hawthorne's effect

This refers to the non-specific effects caused by the knowledge that the research participants have that they are participating in the experimental study. The confounding can be reduced by randomisation, restriction (selecting only participants who have a particular range of values of a potential confounder, e.g. education, social class) and matching. Statistical control of confounding involves two methods: stratified analysis and multivariate analysis using regression.

Bias towards the centre: participants avoid extreme responses and stick to the middle.

Halo effect: this is the observer's error where one judgement is carried over from another. It is a psychological tendency of people to judge others on the basis of a single trait of which they approve but they also conclude that the person must have other attractive traits.

Extreme responding: the participants always agree or disagree with the questions.

184. E Orbitofrontal tumours

Impulsivity with behavioural disinhibition is due to orbitofrontal tumours. There are personality changes, mood lability, irritability, lack of insight with poor judgement, social inappropriateness with immoral language, inappropriate sexuality and tactless gaiety.

185. C Dorsolateral prefrontal convexity tumours

There is apathy and lack of spontaneity, along with abulia, reduced planning ability, psychomotor retardation, impaired concentration, attention and motor impersistence. The symptoms mimic depressive illness.

186. A Anterior cingulate tumours

They cause akinetic mutism.

187. H RD Laing

He was one of the most prominent figures in the anti-psychiatry movement. He challenged the diagnostic labels and the medical model of mental illnesses. He was a Scottish psychiatrist who wrote extensively on mental illness, in particular the experience of psychosis.

188. A Benedict Morel

In 1860, he observed young men being affected by a mental disorder that eventually led to reduced mental functioning and disability. He used the term 'démence precoce' to describe it. As time progressed, it was realised that démence precoce didn't necessarily affect only young adults or lead to mental deterioration. In 1908, Eugene Bleuler coined the term 'schizophrenia' for this recognised disorder.

189. F Karl Ludwig Kahlbaum

In 1874, he first described catatonia as a disorder of unusual motor symptoms. He studied and described the natural course of the symptoms of catatonia as a disorder. Motor immobility (holding rigid postures), motor hyperactivity, mutism, etc. are characteristic features.

Answers: EMIs

190. E John Cade

Lithium was initially introduced to treat bladder stones and gout in the mid-nineteenth century. In the later part of that century, it was shown to be helpful in depression. In the 1940s, lithium chloride was unsuccessfully used to replace sodium chloride for hypertensive patients. John Cade reported its successful use in mania and, later on in the 1950s and 1960s, Mogans Schou demonstrated short-term prophylactic efficacy in bipolar 1 disorder.

191. D Disqualifying the positive

See **Table 1.7** for explanation.

192. I Selective abstraction

See **Table 1.7** for explanation.

193. B Catastrophising

See **Table 1.7** for explanation.

Table 1.7 Cognitive distortions	
Arbitrary inference	Jumping to conclusions
	A person quickly draws a conclusion without the requisite evidence
	Interpreting situations incorrectly by drawing unjustified conclusions
Catastrophising	Magnification
	Blowing things out of proportion
	Focusing on the worst possible outcome
	Common in panic
Dichotomous thinking	All or nothing thinking
	Black or white thinking
	Failure to see the middle ground or grey area
Disqualifying the positive	Failing to acknowledge positive events or aspects of a situation
	Common in depression
Magical thinking	Common in obsessive–compulsive disorder
	For example, because I thought about death, something bad will happen to someone I love
Minimisation	Giving less importance to a situation/issue than it deserves
Overgeneralisation	Unfairly generalising an occurrence from one situation to other situations to which it may not apply
Personalisation	Attributing outcomes or events to oneself when external factors are also of importance
Selective abstraction	Detail is taken out of context and believed while everything else is ignored
	Acknowledgement of one aspect of a situation while ignoring others
	Picking out a single negative and dwelling on it while ignoring the rest
	For example, depressive negative selection

194. E Moderate depression

According to NICE guidelines, young people should not be offered medication for mild depression. For moderate-to-severe depression, fluoxetine should be offered/considered along with psychological therapies. Sertraline and citalopram are second-line drugs. Paroxetine, venlafaxine, tricyclic antidepressants and St John's wort should not be prescribed.

195. G Severe ADHD without co-morbidity

According to NICE guidelines, drug treatment should be offered in school-age children and young people with severe ADHD. Methylphenidate should be considered for ADHD with and without co-morbid conditions such as conduct disorder. Atomoxetine should be considered if methylphenidate has been ineffective or if the young person is intolerant of the drug.

196. A Acute mania

For treatment of children and young people with acute mania, medication management is similar to that in adults except that they should be started at low doses. Height, weight and prolactin levels should be checked at the initial presentation. Olanzapine, risperidone and quetiapine are the options available. It should be noted that lithium is the only drug with current marketing authorisation in the UK for bipolar disorder in patients aged between 12 and 18 years.

197. E Lesch–Nyhan syndrome

Children with the Lesch–Nyhan syndrome show verbal and physical aggression. However, a more characteristic problem, which is resistant to management, is self-injurious behaviour; this affects >85% of these children. Most prominent self-injurious behaviours include biting the lips, the inside of the mouth and the fingers. Other common self-injurious behaviours include thumping of the ears and face, and hitting the head against objects. Although in some cases these behaviours start in adolescence, in most cases they start between the ages of 2 and 3½ years. It is reported in some cases that self-injurious behaviours reduce in frequency and severity after the age of 10.

198. F Prader–Willi syndrome

The behavioural phenotype associated with the Prader–Willi syndrome has been described consisting of abnormalities in speech, sleep and behaviour, along with a specific pattern of cognitive impairment in which individuals show relatively intact visuospatial skills associated with reduced short-term memory and greater loss of memory over time.

Speech abnormalities, including articulation disorder, abnormal syntax among others, have been described.

Sleep abnormalities, including excessive daytime sleepiness, initial insomnia, sleep-onset REM and hyperventilation during REM sleep, have been reported.

A behaviour syndrome consisting of motor slowness, skin picking, sleepiness, ritualistic behaviour, impulsive talk and stubbornness has been described.

199. A Angelman's syndrome

This is also known as the 'happy puppet syndrome'. Angelman's syndrome is characterised by severe learning disability, jerky limb movements associated with abnormal gait and inappropriate bouts of laughter. Most affected children lack speech. Other characteristic clinical features include epilepsy (about 86%) and/or and abnormal EEG, tongue thrusting, hand flapping and mouthing behaviour.

Typical facial features associated with this syndrome consist of long face and prominent jaw, a wide mouth and widely spaced teeth, thin upper lip, midfacial hypoplasia, deep-set blue eyes, blonde hair, flat occiput and microcephaly.

200. G Rett's syndrome

In a postal questionnaire survey of 107 families who rated behaviours among their children with Rett's syndrome, episodes of low mood were reported in 70%, brief episodes of mood changes in 67% and sustained mood changes in 9%. They also reported episodes of anxiety with hyperventilation, screaming, self-injury, a frightened expression and general distress, precipitated by sudden noises, certain music, strange people or places, changes in routine and excessive environmental activity. Self-injurious behaviour may occur in 40–50% of affected girls and is often associated with abnormal hand movements including biting and chewing of the fingers and hands. More severe self-injury may involve hand-to-hand banging, hand-to-object banging, hair pulling, scratching and head banging. Sleep problems, including laughing at night, may affect up to 74% of cases. Many girls also manifest autistic features and between 59 and 72% develop epileptic seizures by age 5.

Chapter 2

Mock Exam: 2

Questions: MCQs

For each question, select one answer option

ORGANISATION AND DELIVERY OF PSYCHIATRIC SERVICES

1. Which one of the following is correct concerning ECT clinic and facilities standards, according to the Electroconvulsive Therapy Accreditation Service (ECTAS)?

    A   The clinic must adhere to the Trust infection policy standards
    B   The clinic must have a minimum of two rooms
    C   ECT treatment is visible from the waiting area
    D   The same space can be used for both the waiting room and recovery room
    E   The treatment room can be used as a staff office when necessary

2. Which of the following is an indicator of positive response to ECT in the treatment of depression?

    A   Automatic negative thoughts
    B   Inability to tolerate oral medication
    C   Moderate to severe depression response to medication
    D   Psychomotor agitation
    E   Puerperal psychosis

3. Which of the following is a contraindication for repetitive transcranial magnetic stimulation (rTMS)?

    A   History of manic behaviour
    B   History of suicidal attempts
    C   History of violent behaviour
    D   Myocardial infarction
    E   Stroke

4. The clinical indications for deep brain stimulation include:

    A   Agoraphobia
    B   Anorexia nervosa
    C   Bipolar affective disorder
    D   Depression
    E   Schizophrenia

5. A 24-year-old female patient was recently admitted to the ward with a history of psychotic symptoms over the last 7 days. These were not related to alcohol or substance misuse. Her

symptoms completely remitted without medication. She has good support from her family. You are an ST4 Trainee in psychiatry working in acute inpatient unit and have discharged the patient home. She wants to know whether she can resume driving her car. Your advice would be:

- A The patient may continue driving and need not inform the DVLA as this is an acute and transient psychotic disorder which has remitted spontaneously.
- B The patient may continue driving but should inform the DVLA as this is an acute and transient psychotic disorder which has remitted spontaneously.
- C The patient should stop driving for at least 1 month and inform the DVLA as this is an acute and transient psychotic disorder.
- D The patient should stop driving for at least 6 months and inform the DVLA as this is an acute and transient psychotic disorder.
- E The patient should stop driving for at least 3 months and inform the DVLA as this is an acute and transient psychotic disorder.

6. Which one of the following statements pertaining to the Mental Health Act 1983 (amended 2007) is correct?

- A A course of ECT can be administered at the discretion of the responsible clinician under the Mental Health Act even if the patient refuses ECT.
- B A patient can be detained for up to 72 hours by the responsible clinician only under section 5(2) of the Mental Health Act
- C It is the responsibility of local social services to provide appropriate care under section 117 of the Mental Health Act
- D It is the responsibility of the mental health services to make sure that approved mental health professionals (AMHPs) are available to carry out appropriate duties and responsibilities.
- E Only psychiatrists can act as responsible clinicians

7. Which of the following is the core feature of 'duty to warn'?

- A Clear risk of serious harm to an identifiable person or group of persons
- B Duty to inform police
- C Duty to inform the neighbours of the intended victims
- D Duty to maintain the patient's autonomy
- E Duty to observe complete confidentiality

RESEARCH METHODS, STATISTICS, CRITICAL REVIEW AND EVIDENCE-BASED PRACTICE

8. ESEMeD was conducted in six countries in Europe and was started in 2000. What does ESEMeD stand for?

- A Early Signs Emerging in Mental Disorders
- B Early Symptoms in Emotional and other Mental Disorders
- C Emerging Signs in Emotional Mental health Disorders
- D European Study of Emergence of Mental Disorders
- E European Study of the Epidemiology of Mental Disorders

9. Which of the following statements about the ESEMeD study is correct?

- A Age range for participants in the study was 16–54 years.
- B It was a cross-sectional study.
- C Patients receiving psychological therapy were not considered, only those on medication.
- D Patients were assessed in inpatient units.
- E Questionnaires were based on SCAN.

10. Which of the following statements about EURODEP studies is correct?
    A   The age of the participants ranged from 18 years to 75 years.
    B   Data were collected from nine centres in Europe to compare prevalence of depression diagnosis.
    C   Depressive symptoms were unrelated to patients attending church or taking part in other religious practices.
    D   India was included in the study.
    E   No significant differences in rates of depression were found between various centres.

11. The IPSS study was conducted in patients with schizophrenia. What does IPSS stand for?
    A   International Pilot Schizophrenia prevention Study
    B   International Pilot Study of Schizophrenia
    C   International Prevalence of Schizophrenia Study
    D   International Prevalence Study of Schizophrenia
    E   International Prevention Study of Schizophrenia

12. You designed a rating scale to study depression in the general population, using the scale in 500 members of a general population. You used the Montgomery–Asberg depression rating scale (MADRS) as a gold standard scale for depression. You had tried to establish the validity of the new scale against an established test. What is this known as?
    A   Concurrent validity
    B   Content validity
    C   Convergent validity
    D   Incremental validity
    E   Predictive validity

13. Which of the following is a characteristic feature of a gaussian distribution?
    A   It is dumbbell shaped.
    B   The mean is greater than the median.
    C   The mode is greater than the mean.
    D   The tails of the curve touch the horizontal axis.
    E   The values continue up to infinity.

14. In analysing study data, the investigator found that the variance is 81 and sample size 9. What is the standard error of the mean?
    A   1
    B   2
    C   3
    D   6
    E   9

15. Which of the following statistical techniques is used to measure interrater reliability?
    A α statistics
    B β statistics
    C   k statistics
    D λ statistics
    E ω statistics

16. In a skewed sample, which of the following is the best measure of central tendency?
    A   Interquartile range
    B   Mean
    C   Median

D   Mode
E   Standard deviation

17. Which of the following is a continuous variable?

    A   IQ of students in a classroom
    B   Men and women in a residential home
    C   Number of episodes of relapse experienced by patients over a lifetime
    D   Number of patients admitted to an inpatient unit in 1 year
    E   Socioeconomic status of patients attending a clinic

18. The research team in Bedford designed a scale to measure psychosis in the general population. The prevalence of psychosis in this population was 4%. The sensitivity and specificity were 0.8 and 0.9, respectively. What is the post-test probability of psychosis in a person with a positive test?

    A   0.13
    B   0.24
    C   0.33
    D   0.44
    E   0.55

19. Which of the following statements about a receiver operating characteristic (ROC) analysis curve is correct?

    A   A test that perfectly discriminates between the two groups would yield a 'curve' that coincided with the left and top sides of the plot.
    B   A test that perfectly discriminates between the two groups would give a straight line from the bottom left corner to the top right corner.
    C   The diagnostic accuracy of a test is given by the area on the left and top sides of the ROC curve.
    D   The ROC has sensitivity values plotted on the x axis.
    E   The ROC has specificity values plotted on the y axis.

20. What is the range of a correlation coefficient?

    A   0–1
    B   0–1000
    C   −1 to +1
    D   1–100
    E   −infinity to +infinity

21. Clinical psychologists developed a new 10-item scale to screen depression in the general population. To check its reliability they divided it into two subscales of five items each and compared their results. What is the statistics measure that is useful in this condition known as?

    A   Cohen's k coefficient
    B   Cronbach's α coefficient
    C   Cronbach's β coefficient
    D   Cronbach's ω coefficient
    E   Wilks' λ coefficient

22. Which of the following statements about the null hypothesis is correct?

    A   The null hypothesis is directional in expressing relationships.
    B   The null hypothesis is used to nullify the difference that arises between two populations in research.
    C   The null hypothesis refers to samples or a particular member of a set in the research study.
    D   The null hypothesis states that there is no difference between two populations.
    E   There will not be any difference between two sample means even when they come from the same population.

Questions: MCQs

23. A study was conducted to assess the extrapyramidal side effects of a new antipsychotic drug in patients with schizophrenia. Many of these patients were smokers and some of them were on anticholinergic drugs. What was the role of the anticholinergic drugs in this study?

    A   Confounder
    B   Dependent variable
    C   Effect modifier
    D   Independent variable
    E   Random variable

24. Which of the following statements about errors in statistics is correct?

    A   The higher the level of significance, the lower the probability of making a type 1 error.
    B   The lower the level of significance, the lower the probability of rejecting the null hypothesis.
    C   A type 1 error is a probability of rejecting a true alternative hypothesis.
    D   A type 2 error is the probability of accepting a true alternative hypothesis.
    E   A type 2 error is denoted by the letter α.

25. You have studied the relationship between IQ scores and psychosis in a general population. Psychosis was studied as a continuous measure of psychotic symptoms rather than a distinct diagnosis. Which of the following statements is accurate?

    A   The association between IQ and psychosis is best described using percentages.
    B   The correlation coefficient can be used to express the association.
    C   If the group with high IQ scores has psychotic symptoms, then high IQ is a risk factor.
    D   Measures of association help us to find the cause of a disorder.
    E   Regression techniques are not used.

Use the following vignette for questions 26–28

You have studied the relationship between cannabis misuse and schizophrenia. You had two sample groups with similar demographic profiles except for smoking cannabis. One of the observations was that patients in both groups had a higher unemployment rate and lower socioeconomic status. The incidence of schizophrenia in the group who smoked cannabis was 10/1000 and the incidence in non-smokers of cannabis was 2/1000.

26. What was the absolute excess risk of developing schizophrenia in the cannabis group of the above study?

    A   0.8
    B   0.08
    C   0.008
    D   0.0008
    E   0.00008

27. What was the relative risk of developing schizophrenia in the cannabis group of the above study?

    A   1
    B   3
    C   5
    D   7
    E   9

28. Suppose, in the above study population, that the prevalence of cannabis misuse was 15/100. What was the population attributable risk?

    A   0.0012
    B   0.012

C   0.024
D   0.12
E   1.2

For each question, select one answer option.

29. Which of the following statements about a normally distributed sample is correct?

    A   Roughly 34% of all scores lie within 1 SD on either side of the mean score.
    B   Roughly 50% of all scores lie within 1 SD on either side of the mean score.
    C   Roughly 68% of all scores lie within 1 SD on either side of the mean score.
    D   Roughly 75% of all scores lie within 1 SD on either side of the mean score.
    E   Roughly 95% of all scores lie within 1 SD on either side of the mean score.

30. Which of the following is a parametric test?

    A   ANOVA
    B   Friedman's test
    C   Kruskal–Wallis test
    D   Whitney–Mann–Wilcoxon test
    E   Wilcoxon's signed rank test

31. Which of the following statements about the Student's *t*-test is correct?

    A   The *t* values are different from the *z* values when there are infinite degrees of freedom.
    B   The tails of *t* distribution are the same as those for a normal distribution.
    C   The tails of *t* distribution inflate directly in relation to the sample number.
    D   The tails of *t* distribution inflate inversely in relation to the sample number.
    E   To apply the Student's *t* test the observations can be dependent.

32. A funnel plot is used to check the existence of bias in a study. What is it called?

    A   Attrition bias
    B   Observer bias
    C   Publication bias
    D   Recall bias
    E   Selection bias

33. A pharmaceutical company conducted a study to evaluate the efficacy of the drug 'Safe' in depression. A group of 100 patients treated with the drug 'Safe' were compared with 100 patients in the standard treatment group, e.g. treatment with imipramine. At the end of a 12-week period, only 60 patients in the 'Safe' group remained in the study; 55 of them scored >50% improvement in the Hamilton Depression Rating (HAM-D) scale. In the imipramine group, 95 patients remained in the study and 50 of them reported an improvement of >50% in HAM-D. Which of the following statements is correct?

    A   All patients who were lost to follow-up would have actually worsened.
    B   Bias as a result of loss of follow-up of patients is called selection bias.
    C   The drug 'Safe' is clinically more effective than imipramine.
    D   The last observation carried forward could be used to correct the error due to loss of follow-up.
    E   Per protocol analysis is the best way to assess the efficacy of the drug 'Safe'.

34. The Yale–Brown Obsessive Compulsive Scale (Y-BOCS) is the gold standard measure of obsessive–compulsive disorder (OCD) symptom severity. In a study, authors examined a sample of 100 patients with a diagnosis of OCD. The results were grouped according to symptom clusters.

These group factors were analysed to study the validity of the scores of Y-BOCS. What type of validity is measured?

A   Construct validity
B   Content validity
C   Criterion validity
D   Face validity
E   Predictive validity

35. You tried to measure the incidence of neurotic symptoms in a general population using a 12-item scale. However, it was noticed that there was a non-systematic distortion or variation of test results. What is this is called?

A   Bias
B   Mistake
C   Non-random error
D   Omission
E   Random error

36. The correlation between two variables is 0.68. What is the coefficient of non-determination?

A   0.35
B   0.46
C   0.54
D   0.63
E   0.72

37. In a study, researchers compared the benefits of quetiapine with those of olanzapine in a group of patients with schizophrenia. Reduction in the PANNS score and improvement in the Global Assessment of Functioning Scale were used as outcome measures. The purpose of the study was to select a drug that can be used economically and safely in clinical practice. Which economic analysis is appropriate?

A   Cost–benefit analysis
B   Cost–consequence analysis
C   Cost-effectiveness analysis
D   Meta-analysis
E   Randomised control trial (RCT)

38. The difference in expected cost of two interventions is divided by the difference in the expected QALYs produced by two interventions. What is this called?

A   Incremental cost–benefit ratio
B   Incremental cost–consequence ratio
C   Incremental cost-effectiveness ratio
D   Incremental cost ratio
E   Incremental cost–utility ratio

Consider the following scenario for answering questions 39–46

A personality disorder questionnaire was designed by the psychology team based at Bedford to screen personality disorders in patients attending primary care services. A study was conducted including 1000 patients from 20 GP surgeries. Initially patients were asked to fill in the questionnaire; subsequently they were interviewed by psychologists involved in the project. The results are shown in **Table 2.1**.

Table 2.1 Results of a personality disorder questionnaire

Personality disorder questionnaire	Structured interview by psychologist		
	Personality disorder diagnosed	Personality disorder not diagnosed	Total
Personality disorder diagnosed	50	110	160
Personality disorder not diagnosed	20	820	840
Total	70	930	1000

39. What is the sensitivity of the personality disorder questionnaire?

    A   0.51
    B   0.61
    C   0.71
    D   0.81
    E   0.91

40. What is the specificity of the personality disorder questionnaire?

    A   0.58
    B   0.68
    C   0.78
    D   0.88
    E   0.98

41. What is the positive predictive value of the personality disorder questionnaire?

    A   0.31
    B   0.61
    C   0.71
    D   0.88
    E   0.97

42. What is the negative predictive value of the personality disorder questionnaire?

    A   0.57
    B   0.67
    C   0.77
    D   0.87
    E   0.97

43. What is the likelihood ratio for a positive test result of the personality disorder questionnaire?

    A   0.32
    B   0.61
    C   1.71
    D   2.88
    E   5.91

44. What is the likelihood ratio for a negative test result of the personality disorder questionnaire?

    A   0.32
    B   0.42
    C   0.52
    D   0.62
    E   0.72

Questions: MCQs

45. What is the prevalence of personality disorder in the study population?

   A   0.03
   B   0.07
   C   1.00
   D   1.04
   E   2.07

46. Which of the following statements about the above study is correct?

   A   The incidence rates of the population are needed to understand predictive values in the context of the population.
   B   The predictive values of a test depend on the incidence of the disease in the population of interest.
   C   The predictive values of a test setting cannot be generalised to a general population.
   D   The sensitivity and specificity of the test cannot be generalised to the general population.
   E   The accuracy of the personality disorder questionnaire is a very useful indicator of the test.

For each question, select one answer option

47. Which of the following is the most appropriate option applicable to Spearman's correlation coefficient?

   A   The data are of normal distribution.
   B   It can be used to test linear associations between two continuous variables.
   C   It is calculated by using the ranks of data observations.
   D   It is used when the two variables being examined are numerical and continuous in nature.
   E   The data are not discrete or ordinal.

48. In which of the following situations is cost–benefit analysis most appropriate?

   A   When it is desirable to compare an intervention for this condition with an intervention for a different condition
   B   When the effect of both interventions is known to be identical
   C   When the effect of the interventions can be expressed in terms of one main variable
   D   When the effect of the interventions on health status has two or more important dimensions
   E   When the effects of both interventions is known to be non-identical

49. A new drug was evaluated against an old drug in terms of the likelihood of bringing about some measure of clinical improvement in a trial of 100 participants with 50 in each group

   Table 2.2 Evaluation of new drug against old drug

Drug	Improved	Not improved	Total
New drug	40	10	50
Old drug	30	20	50
Total	70	30	100

   What is the odds ratio of clinical improvement calculated from **Table 2.2**?

   A   2.63
   B   2.67
   C   6.27
   D   7.21
   E   26.7

50. Which of the following statements about minimisation is correct?
    A Each participant is allocated to the control group.
    B It causes the most imbalance to overall distribution.
    C It involves identifying every prognostic factor in a trial and then applying a weighting system to one of them.
    D It is the most commonly used adaptive method of randomisation.
    E Minimisation is performed in order to shift the balance of distribution of the most important prognostic factor.

51. Which of the following statements about observational methods is correct?
    A Observational methods (covert and overt) are seldom used in the area of health management to identify areas of weakness and possible strategies for healthcare management.
    B Observational methods allow qualitative researchers to assess human behaviours and interactions first hand, along with the impact that these behaviours may have on the subject of interest.
    C Observational methods are best suited for quantitative research questions that are loaded with behavioural or procedural issues.
    D Qualitative researchers arguably embark on covert observational methods to counteract observation bias.
    E The major advantage of observation method is that the very presence of an observer can alter people's behaviour.

52. Which of the following statements about reliability is correct?
    A Content or sampling reliability is the completeness of assessment of the phenomenon.
    B Intrarater reliability is the extent to which one rater is unstable over time.
    C Reliability cannot be quantified as a correlation coefficient.
    D Simple correlations are a satisfactory measure of reliability of a scale, whether these are calculated as the correlation between two halves or the average of all the correlations among the items.
    E Split-half scale reliability is when you compare between the four quarters of a scale.

53. Which of the following statements about cross-sectional surveys is correct?
    A Direct contact surveys are more expensive and time-consuming to conduct.
    B Direct contact surveys include self-completed questionnaires, either situational or surveys of records.
    C Results of surveys involving no contact with responders are easier to analyse because of the increased structure that inevitably accompanies such survey responses.
    D The advantages of surveys involving direct contact with responders result because researchers are directly involved, and more information can be gathered from participants than with non-contact form filling.
    E The disadvantage of contact surveys is that researchers may inadvertently influence or even stifle responses during direct contact.

54. Which of the following statements about survival times is correct?
    A The median survival time can be estimated for as long as survival times remain >0.5.
    B The median survival time is usually presented using p values and confidence intervals.
    C The median survival time represents the time taken for participants to experience half the event.
    D Survival times are generally felt to obey a normal distribution.
    E The mean survival time is defined as the duration from the start of a study that coincides with a 0.5 probability of survival.

55. Which of the following refers to the clinical improvement that occurs in study participants as a result of being in a trial?

   A   Confounding
   B   Hawthorne's effect
   C   Placebo effect
   D   Random effect
   E   Vicarious effect

56. In a randomised controlled trial, each participant receives both the intervention and the control treatments, often separated by a washout period of no treatment. What is the name of such a trial?

   A   Cross-over trial
   B   Factorial design trial
   C   Parallel-group comparison trial
   D   Placebo-controlled trial
   E   Within-subject comparison trial

57. Which of the following statements about a highly sensitive test is correct?

   A   It gives a high percentage of false-negative results.
   B   It gives a high percentage of false positives.
   C   It gives a low percentage of false positives.
   D   It gives a low percentage of false-negative results.
   E   The percentages of false positives and false negatives are almost equal.

GENERAL ADULT PSYCHIATRY

58. In a meta-analysis of a study about the effectiveness of prevention in depression, interesting findings were made. Which of the following statements best describes the main finding?

   A   Older people benefited more from a behavioural programme.
   B   Programmes using fewer than three methods performed better.
   C   Programmes not targeting depression can lead to a reduction in the symptoms of depression.
   D   Selective prevention is superior to universal prevention.
   E   Social support programme had a larger effect size.

59. A 54-year-old woman had had bipolar affective disorder for 20 years. When she was assessed by a junior doctor on her presentation to the emergency services, it was noted that she had had several depressive episodes in the past. However, her three hypomanic episodes were closely related to her treatment with antidepressants. What is the type of bipolar disorder?

   A   Bipolar I
   B   Bipolar II
   C   Bipolar III
   D   Bipolar IV
   E   Bipolar V

60. A 37-old-year man with temporal lobe epilepsy attended your outpatient clinic for assessment. He had recently been acting in a strange manner. He would like to learn more about his condition, especially the psychiatric sequelae. What is the prevalence of psychosis in temporal lobe epilepsy?

   A   5–10%
   B   10–15%

C   15–20%
D   20–25%
E   25–30%

61. A 43-year-old man with temporal lobe epilepsy attended your outpatient clinic for assessment. He had been acting in a strange manner lately. He had been feeling depressed for several weeks. Which of the following antidepressants has a lower seizure induction potential?

    A   Monoamine oxidase inhibitors
    B   Noradrenaline and specific serotoninergic antidepressants
    C   Noradrenergic inhibitors
    D   Serotonin–noradrenaline reuptake inhibitors
    E   Tricyclic antidepressants

62. A 29-year-man contracted HIV about 5 years ago. He attended an HIV clinic for regular check-ups. He would like to learn about the psychiatric morbidity of HIV and AIDs, and how they might affect his condition. Which of the following is most probably affected by the presence of psychiatric morbidity?

    A   Compliance with treatment
    B   Decreased risk factors
    C   Increasing immunity
    D   Less risky behaviour
    E   Enabling the patient to engage with services

63. A 36-year-old woman had an emergency caesarean section at 32 weeks due to abruption of the placenta. The newborn child was found to have an intracranial haemorrhage and showed signs of intrauterine growth retardation. The woman later revealed that she had abused illicit drugs while pregnant. Which of the following drugs is most likely to cause such a problem?

    A   Amphetamines
    B   Cannabis
    C   Cocaine
    D   Methadone
    E   Nicotine

64. A 34-year-old woman was considered to have intermittent, uncontrollable, pathological laughter and crying spells. She was reported to be symptom free otherwise. What is the drug of choice for treatment of her condition?

    A   Dopaminergic drugs
    B   Mirtazapine
    C   Selective serotonin reuptake inhibitors
    D   Tricyclic antidepressant
    E   Quinidine

65. The effects of ECT depend on various physiological changes and the physical characteristics of the treatment. Which of the following correlates best with the improvement seen with ECT?

    A   An accurate estimation of seizure threshold
    B   Degree to which the treating dose exceeds the seizure threshold
    C   Length of the observed tonic–clonic activity
    D   Length of bilateral symmetrical EEG seizure activity
    E   Severity of depression before ECT

66. You assessed a 40-year-old man who suspected his wife of being unfaithful. He wanted to understand why he had been feeling this when he could not find any evidence against her. Which of the following statements is most appropriate about morbid jealousy?

A Geographical separation may be necessary to reduce risks.
B It is an ICD-10-recognised diagnosis.
C It is a disorder of the form of thought.
D It is also known as De Clérambault's syndrome.
E It may not be classed as a delusion.

67. A 35-year-old man was arrested on the charge of attempted murder of his neighbour. You gather that he suspected his wife of having an affair with him. Which of the following is most consistent with the known information about morbid jealousy?

A It usually does not affect women.
B It is associated with bipolar affective disorder.
C It is associated with a low self-esteem.
D It is associated with a generalised anxiety disorder.
E Violence is usually directed at the suspected rival.

68. A 24-year-old primipara gave birth to a healthy boy 4 weeks ago. She has been increasingly snappy with her husband. She had a past history of abuse as a child but no past psychiatric history. She was not breastfeeding. What is the most appropriate management under the circumstances?

A A trial of fluoxetine
B A trial of mirtazapine
C Cognitive–behavioural therapy
D Consider admission to local mother-and-baby unit
E Explanation, reassurance and support by a health visitor

69. A 72-year-old depressed man was referred for ECT because he had not been eating or drinking for several days. He had recently lost a significant amount of weight. Which of the following is the least likely to develop as a potential adverse effect of ECT?

A Cardiac arrhythmias
B Epilepsy
C Headache
D Short-term memory impairment
E Shoulder dislocations

70. A 67-year-old man presented with frequent falls, stiffness in his limbs and tremors over the past 2 years. He had been healthy all his life. He was diagnosed with Parkinson's disease. Which of the following psychiatric sequelae is he most likely to develop?

A Dementia
B Depression
C Mania
D Psychosis
E Tics

71. 'Schizophrenia is not so much a diagnosis as a sane response to an insane society which psychiatrists protect via the labelling and segregation of dissenting victims.' Who said this?

A David Cooper
B Erving Goffman
C Michel Foucault
D RD Laing
E Thomas Szaz

72. You work in a rehabilitation team. Your team has developed a package to improve the socio-occupational abilities of the patients under your care. Which of the following rating scales is most appropriate to evaluate this package?

- A   BPRS (Brief Psychiatric Rating Scale)
- B   CGI (Clinical Global Impression)
- C   GHQ (General Health Questionnaire)
- D   PANSS (Positive and Negative Syndrome Scale)
- E   SOFAS (Social and Occupational Functioning Assessment Scale)

73. You work in an inpatient unit for alcohol detoxification. Which of following scales should be your first choice to assess withdrawal symptoms?

- A   AUDIT (Alcohol Use Disorders Identification Test)
- B   CAGE questionnaire
- C   CIWA (Clinical Institute Withdrawal Assessment)
- D   DAST (Drug Abuse Screening Test)
- E   MAST (Michigan Alcohol Screening Test)

74. A 76-year-old woman had a stroke about 6 months ago. She was making slow but steady recovery from it and was able to manage her daily chores with some help from others. Her family would like to know about the psychiatric sequelae of her stroke. Which stroke lesion is primarily associated with post-stroke depression?

- A   Basal ganglia lesions
- B   Cerebral cortical lesions
- C   Left frontal stroke lesions
- D   Right frontal stroke lesions
- E   Subcortical white matter lesions

75. A 53-year-old man was recently diagnosed with moya-moya disease. Recognising that this is a rare condition, he would like to learn about it. Which of the following statements about moya-moya disease is correct?

- A   Familial moya-moya disease is autosomal recessive.
- B   It is a progressive unilateral occlusive disease (mainly the left internal carotid artery) of the cerebral vasculature.
- C   Moya-moya is Japanese for a 'puff of smoke' and describes the appearance of the resultant network of abnormal small collateral vessels seen on MRI of the brain.
- D   There is a higher incidence of elevated thyroid antibodies.
- E   There is medial thickening of the walls of the end-portions of the internal carotid vessels.

76. A 46-year-old woman was diagnosed with epilepsy some time ago. She attended your outpatient clinic for a review. She had recently read about 'forced normalisation' in an information leaflet. She would like to know more about this. Which of the following statements is correct?

- A   Epilepsy is controlled; EEG recordings of these patients are normal during the psychotic episodes. Forced normalisation has been seen only in patients with partial seizures.
- B   Forced normalisation has been seen only in patients with partial seizures.
- C   It has usually been observed following the natural control of epilepsy without the use of antiepileptic drugs.
- D   Psychoses closely linked to seizures are called alternative psychoses.
- E   The psychosis is usually of a paranoid type with a richness of affective symptoms.

77. A 26-year-old man recently sustained a closed head injury in a road traffic accident. He was brought to your outpatient clinic for psychiatric assessment. He had been acting in an aggressive and abrupt manner since the accident. His mother who accompanied him would like to learn more about his condition. Which of the following is a major predictor of aggression after a head injury?

- A   Anticonvulsant drugs
- B   Antisocial behaviour before the head injury

    C   Confusion and disorientation
    D   Epilepsy
    E   Personality change

78. A 55-year-old man with long history of alcohol dependence syndrome attended a memory clinic psychiatric assessment. His wife informed you that his personal hygiene had deteriorated and he had become forgetful over the past 2 years. Which of the following statements about alcohol-related dementia is correct?

    A   Alcohol-related dementia accounts for 2.5% of the dementia population.
    B   Cerebral atrophy is in the dorsofrontal regions.
    C   It contributes to almost 50% of cognitive impairment in mid-adulthood.
    D   The later the onset, the poorer the prognosis.
    E   The prevalence is high in higher socioeconomic areas.

79. A 31-year-old married man with HIV infection attended your clinic for a 3-monthly review. He would like to learn about the long-term implications of his condition. Which of the following statements about the clinical features of HIV-associated dementia is correct?

    A   Early behavioural symptoms include apathy, reduced spontaneity and emotional responsivity.
    B   In the late stages, speech is usually rapid and fluent.
    C   Late motor symptoms include loss of balance and coordination, clumsiness and leg weakness.
    D   Tests of ocular motility do not show interruption of smooth pursuits, and slowing or inaccuracy of saccades.
    E   The onset of HIV-associated dementia is usually sudden.

80. A 42-year-old man with Creutzfeldt–Jakob disease (CJD) attended your clinic for review. His wife would like to learn more about his condition. Which of the following statements about CJD is correct?

    A   About 50% of affected people present with cerebellar ataxia.
    B   Around 20% of patients die within 6 months.
    C   In the acute phase, protein levels are elevated.
    D   The clinical progression is slow and gradual.
    E   The onset is usually in the 45- to 75-year age group.

81. A 32-year-old man was diagnosed with depersonalisation syndrome. Which of the following has been shown to produce a significant improvement in this condition?

    A   Aripiprazole
    B   Combination of clomipramine and antipsychotic drug
    C   Combination of lamotrigine and antidepressant drug
    D   Combination of lamotrigine and antipsychotic drug
    E   Combination of lofepramine and antipsychotic drug

82. A 19-year-old man with anorexia nervosa attended your clinic for a review. He was keen to learn more about his condition. Which of the following statements about anorexia nervosa in men is correct?

    A   Anorexic men tend to have fewer homosexual tendencies than non-anorexic men.
    B   Atypical gender role behaviour increases the risk of anorexia nervosa in men.
    C   Men with anorexia nervosa have normal testicular function.
    D   The outcome for anorexic men is remarkably similar to that for women.
    E   Previous sexual activity is associated with a poor outcome in anorexic men.

83. What is the most common sexual problem seen in men with social phobia?

   A   Delayed ejaculation
   B   Erectile problems
   C   Low sexual desire
   D   Premature ejaculation
   E   Problems with orgasm

84. In which of the following disorders is pathological jealousy a common presentation?

   A   Anxious personality disorder
   B   Dissocial personality disorder
   C   Paranoid personality disorder
   D   Narcissistic personality disorder
   E   Schizotypal personality disorder

85. Which is the best discriminator of narcissistic personality disorder from borderline personality disorder?

   A   Better anxiety tolerance
   B   Better impulse control
   C   Grandiosity
   D   Greater social adjustment
   E   Less frequent suicide attempts

86. A 58-year-old man was admitted to a medical ward with dermatitis in both his hands and diarrhoea. You were asked to assess him because he was getting increasingly confused and irritable. His wife informed you that he had also had memory problems for some time. He scored 22 on the Mini-Mental State Examination (MMSE) and complained of poor sleep. Which of the following investigations is most likely to help reach a definitive diagnosis?

   A   Assessment of vitamin levels
   B   MRI of the brain
   C   Skin biopsy
   D   Stool examination
   E   Urea and electrolytes

87. An 18-year-old male college student presented with depressive symptoms, tiredness, paranoid delusion, abnormal movements, clumsiness and rigidity. He did not have any past psychiatric history. Which of the following is expected to be the most definitive investigation for diagnosis of Wilson's disease?

   A   Blood examination
   B   CSF examination
   C   Liver biopsy
   D   MRI of the brain
   E   Urine examination

88. Which of the following will confirm the diagnosis of Wilson's disease?

   A   Decreased copper in both plasma and urine.
   B   Decreased serum ceruloplasmin and decreased copper in urine
   C   Decreased serum ceruloplasmin and increased copper in urine
   D   Increased serum ceruloplasmin and decreased copper in urine
   E   Increased serum ceruloplasmin and increased copper in urine

OLD AGE PSYCHIATRY

89. Which of the following statements about delirium is correct?

   A   Children are less susceptible to delirium than adults.
   B   In psychiatric wards, delirium tremens is probably the most common form of delirium seen.
   C   Delirium occurs in about 40% of all general medical and surgical inpatients.
   D   Prescription of multiple medicines is not usually a contributing factor in delirium among elderly patients.
   E   Those with pre-existing dementia are not especially vulnerable to developing delirium.

90. A 79-year-old man was diagnosed with Alzheimer's disease about a year ago. He attended the memory clinic for his 6-monthly review. His daughter who accompanied him would like to know about the brain changes in Alzheimer's disease. What are neurofibrillary tangles primarily made up of?

   A   Amyloid
   B   Hirano bodies
   C   Neurons
   D   Tau
   E   Ubiquitin

91. Which of the following is a characteristic feature seen on a SPECT scan in patients with late-onset dementia?

   A   Cortical enlargement
   B   Decreased ventricular size
   C   Increased cerebral blood flow
   D   Posterior parietal cortex sparing
   E   Preserved white matter

CHILD AND ADOLESCENT PSYCHIATRY

92. A 13-year-old girl who has been diagnosed as having a sleep disorder by her GP was brought to your clinic for psychiatric assessment. You arranged for an EEG and explained the findings of sleep spindles and K-complexes to her mother. In which of the following conditions are the characteristic EEG features observed?

   A   Circadian rhythm sleep disorders
   B   Idiopathic hypersomnia
   C   Night terrors
   D   Somnambulism
   E   Stimulant-dependent sleep disorder (stimulant sleep depression)

93. A 5-year-old girl was brought to her GP because she was scared and her sleep had been disturbed since her grandmother died 3 weeks ago. Which of the following statements about typical 5 year olds' understanding of death is correct?

   A   They understand the concept of deterioration of the body.
   B   They do not understand that death is irreversible and universal.
   C   They can give a narrative account of the sequence of events around bereavement.
   D   They understand that death involves permanent separation.
   E   Understanding of irreversibility and universality comes after understanding of causality.

94. A 12-year-old boy was recently diagnosed with a tic disorder. He attended your clinic for a review with his mother. Both of them would like to learn about his condition. Which of the following statements about tic disorders is correct?

   A   Average age of onset is 11 years.
   B   The prevalence of tics in childhood is 1%.
   C   Tics can be voluntarily suppressed by the sufferers.
   D   Tics cannot be reproduced voluntarily by the patient.
   E   Tics tend to be persistent if they remain untreated after diagnosis.

95. A 13-year-old girl was recently admitted to an eating disorder clinic with severe anorexia nervosa. She had refused treatment on an outpatient basis and continues to do so now. Her parents were ambivalent about their involvement in her care. When a child with anorexia nervosa refuses treatment that is deemed essential, what do the National Institute of Health and Care Excellence (NICE) recommend in the UK?

   A   A second opinion from an eating disorders specialist should be considered only as a last resort.
   B   If parents refuse the treatment, the Mental Health Act should be applied.
   C   Parental consent should be relied on in cases of persistent refusal by the patient.
   D   The Children's Act 1989 should be considered under circumstances where parents also refuse treatment.
   E   The Mental Health Act should not be used where parents give their consent.

96. An 8-year-old boy was diagnosed with attention deficit hyperactivity disorder (ADHD) by his GP. He attended your clinic for assessment and management of his condition. His mother would like to learn more about her son's condition, especially management options. Which of the following should be offered as a first-line treatment for severe ADHD?

   A   Behaviour work
   B   CBT
   C   Educational intervention (advice to teachers)
   D   Medication
   E   Psychological intervention

97. An 8-year-old boy was diagnosed with post-traumatic stress disorder (PTSD) by his GP. He attended your clinic for assessment and management of his condition. His mother would like to learn more about her son's condition. Which of the following statements about PTSD in children and adolescents is correct?

   A   About one in five children meets criteria for PTSD after a range of traumas.
   B   Child survivors find it helpful to talk to parents or peers.
   C   Most children are troubled by repetitive and intrusive thoughts about the accident.
   D   Separation difficulties are common in children but not in adolescents.
   E   Vivid dissociative flashbacks are commonly seen.

98. A 14-year-old girl was diagnosed with obsessive–compulsive disorder (OCD) by her GP. She attended your clinic for further assessment and management. She and her mother would like to learn about her condition and how it might affect her life. Which of the following statements about OCD in children and adolescents is correct?

   A   One in five children reports that certain stimuli trigger their rituals.
   B   Boys have an earlier onset than girls.
   C   Childhood-onset OCD typically begins early in childhood.
   D   Compared with adults, pure obsessions are more common in children.
   E   Girls report more obsessions and boys report more compulsions.

99. A 4-year-old boy was recently diagnosed with autism. He attended your clinic for further assessment. His mother who accompanied him would like to learn about his condition and how it might affect his identical twin brother. Which of the following about concordance rate for autism is correct?

    A   Monozygotic rate of 10–15%
    B   Monozygotic rate of 20–30%
    C   Monozygotic rate of 35–55%
    D   Monozygotic rate of 40–60%
    E   Monozygotic rate of 60–90%

100. Which of the following is one of the five outcomes of 'Every child matters' by the Department for Education?

    A   Achieve positive mental health
    B   Attend school
    C   Earn and be economically independent
    D   Eat and live well
    E   Make a positive contribution

101. Child protection is an important matter. In the UK, children are entitled to protection from harmful environments and people. Which of the following statements about British law in relation to children is correct?

    A   A child assessment order lasts 10 days and is not available for use in emergencies.
    B   The National Society for the Prevention of Cruelty to Children (NSPCC) cannot apply for a care order but a local authority can.
    C   Only a local authority can apply for an emergency protection order.
    D   Section 25 allows the child to be placed in secure accommodation if he or she is likely to abscond.
    E   Wardship, in which the court takes parental responsibility, is used when a child's welfare is at risk.

102. It has been found that 90% of young adult delinquents had a conduct disorder as children. What proportion of children with conduct disorder become delinquent young adults with ongoing behaviour problems and disrupted relationships?

    A   20%
    B   40%
    C   60%
    D   80%
    E   90%

103. Which of the following disorders is more common in women than in men?

    A   Asperger's syndrome
    B   Encopresis
    C   Selective mutism
    D   Separation anxiety disorder
    E   Gilles de la Tourette's syndrome

104. A 9-year-old boy with ADHD presented to your clinic for assessment. His mother wanted to learn more about her son's condition. Which of the following statements is about ADHD is correct?

    A   ADHD, compulsive type is one of the three subtypes.
    B   Behavioural strategies are as effective as medication.
    C   Most common overlap of symptoms of ADHD is with anxiety disorders.
    D   The point prevalence of ADHD is about 5%.
    E   Stimulants are contraindicated if co-morbid Gilles de la Tourette's syndrome is present.

LEARNING DISABILITY

105. A 15-year-old boy with learning disability and psychotic symptoms attended your outpatient clinic. His mother, who accompanied him, would like to know about psychotic disorders in people with a learning disability. What is the prevalence of psychotic disorders in this population?

    A   0.1–0.5%
    B   0.5–1%
    C   1–2%
    D   3–3.5%
    E   5–10%

106. A 13-year-old boy was diagnosed with severe learning disability associated with some physical abnormalities. His mother would like to know whether her younger son would be affected with the same condition. Which of the following conditions occurs only in males and is associated with significant learning difficulty?

    A   Duchenne muscular dystrophy (Xp21.2)
    B   Fragile X syndrome
    C   Klinefelter's syndrome
    D   Neurofibromatosis
    E   Turner's syndrome

107. A 14-year-boy was diagnosed with Sanfilippo's syndrome. He attended your outpatient clinic with his mother who wanted to have some information about him. Which of the following statements about Sanfilippo's syndrome is correct?

    A   It is an autosomal dominant disorder.
    B   The prevalence is approximately 1 in 2000.
    C   The prognosis is good, with adults being able to live independently
    D   The clinical features include mild learning disability and somatic features including hair loss.
    E   There is a fault in the breakdown of heparin sulphate.

108. A 39-year-old man with a mild learning disability was brought to A&E because he had recently become psychotic and aggressive. His father who accompanied him would like to know about his condition. Which of the following statements about psychosis in learning-disabled adults is correct?

    A   Catatonic features are common.
    B   Delusional systems tend to be elaborate.
    C   Short-term psychotic states are unusual.
    D   The degree of psychosis tends to be subtle rather than florid.
    E   The prevalence of psychosis is the same as in the general population.

109. A 10-year-old boy diagnosed with a severe learning disability was brought to your outpatient clinic for further assessment. His mother found it very difficult to communicate with him. Which of the following statements about sensory impairment in intellectual disability is correct?

    A   Approximately two-thirds of cases of visual impairment go unnoticed by carers.
    B   Research has shown that 40% of people with severe intellectual disability have visual impairments.
    C   Rubella can cause congenital hearing loss and developmental delay but not visual impairment.
    D   The prevalence of hearing impairment is 10 times higher than in the general population.
    E   Usher's syndrome is a rare cause of deaf–blindness and is associated with psychosis.

110. A 24-year-old man with Down's syndrome diagnosed with OCD was brought to your outpatient clinic for assessment. His care coordinator would like to know more about his condition. Which of the following statements about the most common compulsion seen in adults with learning disability is correct?

A Cleaning
B Hair pulling
C Hand washing
D Nail biting
E Ordering

111. A 6-year-old girl was diagnosed with severe leaning disability. Her mother blamed herself for her daughter's condition. You tried to explain the possible causes of such conditions. Which of the following is the most common single cause of severe generalised learning difficulty?

A Birth trauma
B Down's syndrome
C Fragile X syndrome
D Head injury
E Neonatal infection

112. Which of the following is an X-linked recessive condition?

A Fragile X syndrome
B Hunter's syndrome
C Hurler's syndrome
D Neurofibromatosis
E Phenylketonuria

FORENSIC PSYCHIATRY

113. Which of the following statements about domestic abuse in the UK is correct?

A One in ten women experiences domestic abuse at some point in her life.
B A domestic violence perpetrator's sense of entitlement is an attempt to compensate for poor self-image.
C Group work for perpetrators is preferred because it reduces their isolation.
D Most perpetrator programmes are influenced by feminist theory.
E Women most at risk are aged >50 years.

114. A 26-year-old man was charged with indecent exposure (exhibitionism) and appeared in court. His defence lawyer requested a psychiatric report on him. The lawyer would like to learn about various aspects of people who commit indecent exposure. Which of the following statements about indecent exposure is correct?

A It is rare for exhibitionists to show other paraphilias.
B The majority of male first offenders do not reoffend after their conviction.
C Personality characteristics include being an extrovert.
D The use of anti-libidinal drugs is not appropriate in this group.
E They usually make attempts to enter a relationship with the victim.

115. A 30-year-old nurse was assessed after being charged with physical abuse of her 5-year-old son. Which of the following statements about Munchausen's syndrome by proxy is correct?

A The children do not have a genuine underlying illness.
B Male victims are more common than female victims.

C   The mortality rate in children is approximately 20%.
D   The mothers have a high incidence of somatoform disorders.
E   Most families have serious marital problems.

116. Which of the following categories of maternal filicide is the most common in prison?

   A   Killing unwanted children
   B   Mentally ill mothers
   C   Mercy killing
   D   Neonaticides
   E   Retaliating mothers

117. A 50-year-old man serving a sentence for a sexual offence is to be released soon. Which of the following is associated with a decreased risk of reoffending?

   A   Absence of psychiatric illness
   B   High number of previous sexual offences
   C   High scores on psychopathy scales
   D   Presence of violent sexual fantasies
   E   Previous criminal history

118. Which of the following statements about assessment of risk of violence in a mentally disordered person is correct?

   A   Actuarial tools are of no practical help to the clinicians.
   B   Clinical experience is the most reliable guide.
   C   Contextual variables should be ignored.
   D   Structured professional judgement has been shown to be a valid approach.
   E   Using the HCR-20 guarantees an estimate that is free of bias.

119. Which of the following statements about suicides in prison is correct?

   A   Antecedents are clearly apparent in those who are about to commit suicide.
   B   It is more common in sentenced prisoners than remand prisoners.
   C   It is the second most common cause of death in prisoners.
   D   It is usually done by overdose.
   E   The rate is approximately eight to nine times that found in the general population.

SUBSTANCE MISUSE/ADDICTIONS

120. A 19-year-old university student was brought to A&E after a night out with his friends. He had consumed a large quantity of LSD and cannabis. Which of the following is the preferred treatment for hallucinogen intoxication?

   A   Diazepam
   B   Haloperidol
   C   Sedation
   D   Supportive counselling
   E   Talking down the patient

121. A 30-year-old woman with a history of alcohol abuse came to the clinic with her 1-year-old daughter who might have fetal alcohol syndrome. Which of the following is a characteristic feature of fetal alcohol syndrome?

   A   Intellectual disability
   B   Macrocephaly

C   Renal dysfunction
D   Seizures
E   Tall stature

122. Which of the following is the correctly matched half-life of misused substances?

A   Amphetamine: 2 min
B   Cannabis: 2 hours
C   Heroin: 12 hours
D   Methadone: 36 hours
E   Diazepam: 7 days

123. A 30- year-old pregnant woman has been dependent on heroin for the last 2 years. She is expected to deliver a baby in 2 days. Which of the following statements describes what is likely to happen in the newborn baby?

A   Gastrointestinal disturbances are uncommon withdrawal symptoms.
B   It is likely that withdrawal symptoms will be evident within 1 hour of birth.
C   There is a 70% chance that the neonate will show no withdrawal symptoms.
D   The onset of withdrawal symptoms may begin up to 10 days after birth.
E   The baby is likely to be lethargic with reduced muscle tone.

PSYCHOTHERAPY

124. A 29-year-old woman diagnosed with borderline personality disorder attended your outpatient clinic for a review of her care plan. She asked why she was not making any progress. Which of the following defence mechanisms is found most frequently in patients with borderline personality disorder?

A   Denial
B   Displacement
C   Projection
D   Repression
E   Splitting

125. A 35-year-old man with a psychotic disorder attended your outpatient clinic for a review. He complained of some problem with his eyesight. Which of the following syndromes is associated with visual impairments?

A   Capgras' syndrome
B   Charles Bonnet syndrome
C   Cotard's syndrome
D   Couvade's syndrome
E   De Clérambault's syndrome

126. A 27-year-old man was convicted of a serious criminal offence. The court had ordered a psychiatric report. While examining him, you were not sure whether or not he has a mental disorder. You believed that he appeared to be mimicking his view of what constituted a severe mental disorder. Which of the following syndromes best describes this presentation?

A   Briquet's syndrome
B   Diogenes' syndrome
C   Ganser's syndrome
D   Othello's syndrome
E   Munchausen's syndrome

127. According to Yalom, universality, altruism, catharsis and existential factors are therapeutic factors in which type of psychological therapy?

    A   Cognitive-behavioural therapy
    B   Dialectical behaviour therapy
    C   Group psychotherapy
    D   Individual psychodynamic psychotherapy
    E   Systemic family therapy

128. A 37-year-old woman presenting frequently to her GP was considered to be feigning a number of physical symptoms, which included back pain and upper limb symptoms that she said had prevented her from carrying out her usual daily work in the family home. There did not seem to be any specific external incentives for her behaviour. What is the most likely psychiatric diagnosis?

    A   Factitious disorder
    B   Hypochondriasis
    C   Hysterical conversion
    D   Malingering
    E   Somatisation disorder

129. Which of the following is a disorder of sexual preference according to ICD-10?

    A   Bestiality (zoophilia)
    B   Homosexuality
    C   Masturbation
    D   Transvestism
    E   Voyeurism

130. A 25-year-old man presented with a delusional belief that he was infested with parasites. He reported 'bugs' crawling under his skin. There was no evidence of any skin infection. A diagnosis of Ekbom's syndrome was made. Which of the following statements is correct?

    A   It is more common in women than in men.
    B   It is rare with a prevalence of <1%.
    C   Prevalence reduces with age.
    D   Symptoms are relieved with rest.
    E   Symptoms become more pronounced in the evenings.

Questions :EMIs

RESEARCH METHODS, STATISTICS, CRITICAL REVIEW AND EVIDENCE-BASED PRACTICE

Theme: Concepts in critical appraisal

Options for questions: 131–133

A   Confounder
B   Content validity
C   Intention-to-treat analysis
D   Positive predictive value
E   Relative risk
F   Specificity
G   Type 2 error

For each of the following descriptions, select the single most appropriate response. Each option may be used once, more than once or not at all.

131. In a study to understand the relationship between young people with mental illness and crime, researchers found that drug use was associated with both mental illness and acquisitive offending.

132. A test, when administered to 50 people with suspected agoraphobia, identified the 10 people who did not have the illness. This was later confirmed by clinical interview.

133. During a randomised controlled trial with 200 participants over 4 months, 40 dropped out. The scores for the final outcome point were imputed for the 40 participants.

Theme: Statistical data

Options for questions: 134–136

A   Binary data
B   Continuous data
C   Interval data
D   Nominal data
E   Ordinal data
F   Ratio data

For each of the following descriptions, select the single most appropriate response. Each option may be used once, more than once or not at all.

134. Dead or alive

135. Social class

136. Fahrenheit scale

GENERAL ADULT PSYCHIATRY

Theme: Culture-bound syndromes

Options for questions: 137–139

A   Amok
B   Ataque de nervios
C   Bouffée délirante
D   Brain fag
E   Dhat
F   Koro

G   Latah
H   Piblokto
I   Susto
G   Zar

For each of the following cases, select the single most appropriate diagnosis. Each option may be used once, more than once or not at all.

137. A 32-year-old man from the Arctic region had an abrupt dissociative episode characterised by tearing off of clothing, breaking furniture, shouting obscenities and extreme excitement for about half an hour, followed by a seizure. He did not remember the episode later on.

138. A 40-year-old Nepalese man complained of weakness and exhaustion and believed that this was the result of masturbation.

139. A 27-year-old West African man developed a sudden outburst of agitation, aggression, confusion and psychomotor excitement. He also had paranoid ideas and visual hallucinations.

Theme: Prion diseases

Options for questions: 140–142

A   Chronic wasting disease
B   Creutzfeldt–Jakob disease
C   Gerstmann–Sträussler–Scheinker syndrome
D   Kuru
E   Scrapie
F   Transmissible mink encephalopathy

For each of the following cases, select the single most appropriate diagnosis. Each option may be used once, more than once or not at all.

140. It includes chronic cerebellar ataxia accompanied by pyramidal features, with dementia occurring later in a much more prolonged clinical course.

141. It reached epidemic proportions among the Fore language group in Papua New Guinea and was transmitted by ritual cannibalism.

142. It is a rapidly progressive multifocal dementia, usually with myoclonus.

OLD AGE PSYCHIATRY

Theme: Psychiatric presentations in elderly people

Options for questions: 143–145

A   Capgras' syndrome
B   Charles Bonnet syndrome
C   Dementia with Lewy bodies
D   Diogenes' syndrome
E   Fregolli's syndrome
F   Frontotemporal dementia
G   Möbius' syndrome
H   Paraphrenia
I   Temporal lobe epilepsy

For each of the following cases, select the single most appropriate diagnosis. Each option may be used once, more than once or not at all.

143. A 74-year-old woman with type 1 diabetes and diabetic retinopathy presented with increased agitation due to seeing small seamen in her bedroom. Her son gave a history of good premorbid functioning, some fluctuating minimal cognitive impairment, which was recent, and the absence of any past psychiatric history.

144. The neighbour of an 81-year-old man called the police because the increasing number of old car parts were filling the man's garden and now encroaching on his own. On approaching the man,

the police found an elderly man presenting with severe self-neglect. On inspection of the house, it was dirty, filled with old newspapers and old car parts from a junkyard, and had signs of vermin infestation.

145. A 67-year-old man developed difficulties with walking. His wife reported some episodes of confusion, but felt that they were variable. She called the GP because he had become increasingly more paranoid, believing that people were taking his money. He was convinced that he could see people coming into his room.

Theme: Diagnosis of dementia

Options for questions: 146–148
A   Alzheimer's dementia
B   Delirium unspecified
C   Depressive peudo-dementia
D   Korsakoff's syndrome
E   Lewy body dementia
F   Normal pressure hydrocephalus
G   Schizophrenia
H   Vascular dementia

For each of the following cases, select the single most appropriate diagnosis. Each option may be used once, more than once or not at all.

146. A 74-year-old man was admitted to the geriatric ward, becoming increasingly aggressive to his wife. He was confused and unable to care for himself. He was found to have an underlying urinary tract infection. After a week of treatment with an antibiotic, his urine was clear and had no other septic focus. He remains confused with gross functional deficits.

147. A 56-year-old engineer began having difficulties at work. He became agitated and his wife reported that he was not the person she had known over the past 20 years. On Addenbrooke's Cognitive Examination – revised (ACE-R), he scored 79/100.

148. An 89-year-old woman was brought to the memory clinic with a history of deteriorating memory over the past 4 months. She had started isolating herself and lost weight. There was some evidence of self-neglect and she had become guarded.

Theme: Treatment of dementia

Options for questions: 149–151
A   Amisulpride
B   Carbamazepine
C   Citalopram
D   Clozapine
E   Donepezil
F   Galantamine
G   Memantine
H   Olanzapine
I   Quetiapine
J   Risperidone
K   Rivastigmine

For each of the following cases, select the single most appropriate treatment. Each option may be used once, more than once or not at all.

149. A 73-year-old man presented with increasing confusion and parkinsonism. He had experienced difficulties with his shopping and paying his bills.

150. An 81-year-old woman with a history of mixed dementia had been on galantamine for the past 1 year. She had barricaded herself in her house, not allowing carers or family in, believing that they were trying to harm her. She stopped eating, thinking that her food was poisoned.

151. A 76-year-old man with a diagnosis of dementia in Alzheimer's disease was started on donepezil. He developed palpitations and bradycardia. Donepezil was stopped and he was tried on rivastigmine and again became dizzy with bradycardia. He still lived in his own home and functioned very well.

FORENSIC PSYCHIATRY

Theme: Sex ratio of mental disorders

Options for questions: 152–154

A   Autistic disorders
B   Depression (postpubertal)
C   Depression (prepubertal)
D   Hyperactivity disorder
E   School refusal
F   Selective mutism
H   Specific phobias
I   Tic disorders

For each of the following cases, select the most appropriate diagnoses according to further instructions. Each option may be used once, more than once or not at all.

152. Marked male excess [select THREE options]

153. Male and females approximately equal [select THREE options]

154. Marked female excess [select TWO options]

CHILD AND ADOLESCENT PSYCHIATRY

Theme: Developmental milestones

Options for questions: 155–157

A   0–1 month
B   1–3 months
C   3–5 months
D   5–10 months
E   10–18 months
F   18–36 months
G   3–5 years
H   5–7 years
I   7–10 years

For each of the following cases, select the single most appropriate response. Each option may be used once, more than once or not at all.

155. Smiles spontaneously

156. Shy with strangers

157. Dry by day

GENERAL ADULT PSYCHIATRY

Theme: Epileptic foci and respective symptoms

Options for questions: 158–161

A   Frontoparietal lobe
B   Left frontal lobe focus
C   Left parietal lobe focus
D   Left temporal lobe focus
E   Right frontal lobe focus
F   Right parietal lobe focus
G   Right temporal lobe focus
H   Temporal lobe epilepsy (TLE)

For each of the following cases, select the single most appropriate diagnosis. Each option may be used once, more than once or not at all.

158. Speech automatism, and recurrent, irrelevant and emotionally toned utterances

159. Transient dysphasia

160. Compulsion to think on restricted topics such as religiosity, eternity, death

161. The whole episode from the patient's past life is relived in a brief period of time as a complex organised experience; also called panoramic memory

OLD AGE PSYCHIATRY

Theme: Cognitive examination

Options for questions: 162–164

A   Three-item recall
B   Seven-item recall
C   Attention and concentration
D   Clock-drawing test
E   Cognitive estimates
F   Frontal lobe test
G   Motor fluency test
H   Occipital lobe test
I   Parietal lobe test
J   Temporal lobe test
K   Verbal fluency test

For each of the following cases, select the single most appropriate cognitive test. Each option may be used once, more than once or not at all.

162. Constructional apraxia and left-right disorientation are localised to this lobe.

163. Serial 7s tests this cognitive domain.

164. The go–no-go test assesses function in this lobe.

SUBSTANCE MISUSE/ADDICTIONS

Theme: Complications with use of illicit drugs

Options for questions: 165–167

A   Alcohol
B   Amphetamines
C   Cannabis
D   LSD
E   Magic mushrooms
F   Methylphenidate
G   Opioids
H   Temazepam

For each of the following diagnosis, select the single most appropriate offending drug. Each option may be used once, more than once or not at all.

165. Amotivational syndrome

166. Morbid jealousy

167. Neonatal abstinence syndrome

FORENSIC PSYCHIATRY

Theme: Psychiatric defence for criminal proceedings in UK

Options for questions: 168–171

A Diminished responsibility
B Infanticide
C Insane automatism
D Not fit to plead
E Not guilty by reason of insanity
F Sane automatism
G Suicide pact

For each of the following cases, select the single most likely psychiatric court defence, which may be used once, more than once or not at all.

168. A 33-year-old man beheaded his neighbour. For some time, he had experienced a system of delusional beliefs supported by auditory hallucinations that he was God. Although he knew the nature and quality of the act of killing, he did not know that it was wrong. He believed that, as the neighbour was the devil, his action was justified.

169. A 50-year-old accountant was depressed after being charged with the murder of his wife. His illness prevented him from adequately instructing his legal advisers.

170. A 32-year-man with epilepsy was admitted to hospital after 2 grand-mal fits. He was confused, paranoid and hallucinating. After a minor seizure, he significantly assaulted a fellow patient on the ward.

171. A 37-year-old woman was arrested for killing her sister. For some weeks before this incident, she had experienced a delusional belief that her sister undermined her work and social status. She had command auditory hallucinations telling her to kill her sister. At the police interview, she told them that she knew killing was wrong.

RESEARCH METHODS, STATISTICS, CRITICAL REVIEW AND EVIDENCE-BASED PRACTICE

Theme: Statistical tests of significance

Options for questions: 172–174

A ANOVA test
B Fisher's exact test
C Freidman's test
D Kruskal Wallis test
E Mann–Whitney U-test
F McNemar's test
G Wilcoxon's signed rank test

For each of the following descriptions, select the single most appropriate statistical test. Each option may be used once, more than once or not at all.

172. This is used in comparing three or more groups where the data are skewed.

173. This is used in comparing three or more paired samples when data are skewed/discrete numerical/ranked categorical.

174. This is used in comparing three or more groups where the data are normal.

Theme: Hypothesis tests

Options for questions: 175–177

A Bonferroni's correction
B χ^2 test
C Kruskal–Wallis test
D Logistic regression
E Mann–Whitney U-test
F Matched-pair Student's t-test
G McNemar's test
H Wilcoxon's signed rank test

For each of the following descriptions, select the single most appropriate response. Each option may be used once, more than once or not at all.

175. Data can be either nominal or ordinal. The test is used to measure differences between groups across categories.

176. Data can have any distribution. The test is used to test differences in medians of two matched groups.

177. The differences between two groups should be normally distributed. It is used to test differences in means between two groups.

GENERAL ADULT PSYCHITARY

Theme: Neurological symptoms after head injury

Options for questions: 178–180

A Dysphasia
B Dysprosody
C Jargon aphasia
D Post-concussion syndrome
E Reduplicative paramnesia
F Visual agnosia

For each of the following cases, select the single most appropriate diagnosis. Each option may be used once, more than once or not at all.

178. A constellation of symptoms that might result in surprisingly severe disability after a mild head injury.

179. A phenomenon in which the normal rhythms and intonations of speech are lost.

180. Any delusion involving duplication, e.g. that events have been duplicated or that the patient has a second left leg.

RESEARCH METHODS, STATISTICS, CRITICAL REVIEW AND EVIDENCE-BASED PRACTICE

Theme: Features of a diagnostic test

Options for questions: 181–185

A Accuracy
B Likelihood ratio
C Negative predictive value (NPV)
D Positive predictive value (PPV)

E   Reliability
F   Sensitivity
G   Specificity
H   Validity

For each of the following cases, select the single most appropriate feature. Each option may be used once, more than once or not at all.

181. It is about how good the test is at picking up those who have the condition.

182. It is about how good the test correctly excludes people without the condition.

183. It is the probability that he or she has the condition when the test is positive.

184. It is the probability that he or she does not have the condition when the test is negative.

185. It is the proportion of all tests given the correct result.

GENERAL ADULT PSYCHIATRY

Theme: Drug treatment for dementia

Options for questions: 186–190

A   Donepezil
B   Galantamine
C   Haloperidol
D   Memantine
E   Olanzapine
F   Risperidone
G   Rivastigmine
H   Sertraline
I   Trazodone
J   Zopiclone

For each of the following descriptions, select the single most appropriate drug. Each option may be used once, more than once or not at all.

186. It is an antidepressant used as a hypnotic in elderly people.

187. It is the only cholinesterase inhibitor available as a patch used in patients who have swallowing difficulty.

188. It is the only licensed antipsychotic medication for use in behavioural symptoms in dementia.

189. It is the safest cholinesterase inhibitor for patient with pre-existing cardiac problems.

190. It is the only short-acting cholinesterase inhibitor available as a once-daily formulation.

Theme: Mechanisms of action of psychotropic drugs

Options for questions: 191–193

A   Alcohol
B   Cannabis
C   Diazepam
D   γ-Hydroxybutyrate (GHB)
E   Heroin
F   LSD
G   MDMA
H   Nicotine

For each of the following descriptions, select the single most appropriate drug. Each option may be used once, more than once or not at all.

191. This drug releases catecholamine from presynaptic terminals, activating the reward circuit pathway. It is taken up by the serotonin transporter and causes release of large quantities of serotonin, along with inhibiting serotonin synthesis.

192. This drug has an effect similar to other CNS depressants such as barbiturates or ethanol. It is thought that it may enhance GABA circuits through membrane fluidisation.

193. No single molecular target has been identified. However, it is thought that this drug increases ion channel activities in acetylcholine, 5HT3 and GABA type A receptors, and inhibits ion channels of glutamate and calcium.

RESEARCH METHODS, STATISTICS, CRITICAL REVIEW AND EVIDENCE-BASED PRACTICE

Theme: Statistical errors in published research

Options for questions: 194–196

A   Ceiling effect
B   Data dredging
C   Floor effect
D   Mass effect
E   Misused statistical testing
F   Multiple hypothesis testing
G   Order effect
H   Regression to the mean sequential effect

For each of the following descriptions, select the single most appropriate statistical error. Each option may be used once, more than once or not at all.

194. This occurs when a test result is so high that is very unlikely to be able to identify differences between two groups.

195. This is a systematic difference between a first and subsequent assessments.

196. This is stated if any measure is repeated; outliers are likely to tend towards the sample mean owing to measurement error.

Theme: Bias in research studies

Options for questions: 197–200

A   Cognitive bias
B   Experimenter bias
C   Information bias
D   Observer bias
E   Prevalence bias
F   Recall bias
G   Selection bias
H   Social desirability bias

For each of the following cases, select the single most appropriate bias. Each option may be used once, more than once or not at all.

197. This bias occurs whenever subjective factors within an assessor affect the way in which observations are recorded and scored.

198. Bias occurs whenever a characteristic associated with the variable(s) or outcome of a study affects the very probability of being selected for participation in that study.

199. Bias arises from systematic misclassification of data.

200. Bias occurs when sample participants are selected from a specialised setting containing people with a 'special' form of disorder of interest.

Answers: MCQs

1. A The clinic must adhere to the Trust infection policy standards

According to ECTAS standards, the ECT clinic should have a minimum of three rooms (including a pre-treatment, treatment and recovery room). The ECT treatment room should not be visible from the waiting area. The waiting room and recovery rooms are two separate rooms. Similarly, staff office space must be separate from the treatment room.

2. B Inability to tolerate oral medication

The indicators for positive response to ECT include stupor, moderate to severe depression, not responding to medications, puerperal depression, depression with severe self-neglect, diet restriction and nihilistic or paranoid delusions.

3. E Stroke

The other contraindications include epilepsy and brain tumours. Repetitive transcranial magnetic stimulation (rTMS) is a non-invasive and non-convulsive treatment for depression. It takes an advantage of the link between magnetism and electricity, e.g. electric currents generate magnetic fields and vice versa. The electromagnetic induction elicits a focal current in the brain tissues which is strong enough to trigger action potentials in the neurons.

4. D Depression

The deep brain stimulation should be considered as an experimental treatment for depression and obsessive compulsive disorder. The procedure consists of bilateral implantation of electrodes in the brain using stereotactic guidance. This is confirmed by MR scanning. The electrodes are then connected to a generator implanted in the abdomen. Adverse effects include a throbbing or buzzing sensation in the head, nausea and jaw tingling.

5. E Patient should stop driving for at least three months and inform the DVLA as this is an acute and transient psychotic disorder.

In this situation, the patient should stop driving and inform DVLA immediately. DVLA will consider re-licensing once she remains well and stable for a minimum period of three months. She should also comply with the treatment and be free from adverse effect of medication that would impair driving. This should be supported by the treating consultant's report.

6. C It is the responsibility of local social services to provide appropriate care under section 117 of the Mental Health Act.

Under the Mental Health Act 1983 (amended 2007) ECT should be administered only with informed consent of the patient. If the patient refuses, a second opinion from an independent doctor appointed by The Care Quality Commission (England) is required. Under exceptional situations, the responsible clinician may administer emergency ECT under section 62 of the Mental Health Act until a second opinion is obtained.

A voluntary ('informal') mentally ill inpatient can be detained by the responsible clinician or their nominated deputy for a period of up to 72 hours to allow a formal mental health assessment. Patients who are discharged from certain sections of the Mental Health Act are eligible for section 117 arrangements. The local social services have a duty to provide appropriate care under this section, i.e. further treatment related to the condition is free for the patient. It is the responsibility of the local social service authorities to make sure that mental health professionals are available 24 hours a day to carry out duties and responsibilities. Under the Mental Health Act 1983 (amended 2007) any mental health professional could become a responsible clinician, following appropriate training.

7. A A clear risk of serious harm to an identifiable person or group of persons.

Duty to warn refers to the responsibility of a clinician or therapist to breach confidentiality if the patient or other identifiable person is in clear or imminent danger. The confidentiality of the therapeutic relationship is subordinate to the safety of the public and the patients. To justify breach of confidentiality the following questions need to be asked:

- Is there a clear risk to an identifiable person or group of people?
- Is there a risk of serious bodily harm or death?
- Is the victim accessible?
- Is the danger imminent?

If the answer is 'yes' to any of the questions, one is obliged to breach confidentiality.

8. E European Study of the Epidemiology of Mental Disorders.

ESEMeD was conducted in six countries across Europe, namely Belgium, France, Germany, Italy, the Netherlands and Spain. It was initially called the European Study of the Epidemiology of Mental Disorders/Mental Health Disability (ESEMeD/MHEDEA).

9. B It was a cross-sectional study.

ESEMeD investigated the prevalence and associated factors of mental disorders and their effect on health-related quality of life and service usage in the six European countries. The age of participants was ≥18 years. Patients receiving medication and/or psychological therapies were considered in the study. Assessments took place in the community with the help of computer-assisted techniques. Questionnaires were based on the CIDI (Composite International Diagnostic Interview), which is a comprehensive and fully structured diagnostic interview schedule for assessment of mental disorders. The study found that the prevalence estimates of mental disorders were in the highest proportion in Belgium and France and the lowest proportion in Italy and Spain. Co-morbidity of mood and anxiety disorders was frequent in all six countries. However, the use of mental health services was low in all countries and lowest in Italy. Interestingly only 20% of the participants with mental disorders had consulted health services in the preceding year.

10. B Data were collected from nine centres in Europe to compare prevalence of depression diagnosis.

The age of the participants was >65 years. Depressive symptoms were noted to be fewer in participants attending church or taking part in other religious practices. The prevalence of depression differed between countries. The highest level of depression was seen in Munich (23.6%) and the lowest in Iceland (8.8%). The UK was part of the study. The EURO-D scale was used in 14 population-based surveys. The depression score tended to increase with age, unlike the prevalence rates of depression. The study showed that depression was common in older people and treatment opportunities were missed.

11. B International Pilot Study of Schizophrenia

IPSS was a large epidemiological pilot study involving nine countries. It was conducted in the 1970s to assess the feasibility of an epidemiological study on schizophrenia and functional psychiatric disorders throughout the world. It demonstrated that standardised assessment tools could be developed for such large-scale studies. An important finding on schizophrenia was that its prevalence was uniform worldwide. However, the outcomes, both clinical and social or both together, were better in developing countries compared with developed countries. The study was unable to identify a variable that was responsible for the notable difference in the outcomes.

12. A Concurrent validity

This refers to the level of agreement between the findings of a new test and the findings of an established test. In this question, a new scale was tried against a gold standard scale – MADRS. Content validity refers to the type of validity that looks into whether the test or measure actually assesses all the domains of the disorder, e.g. a scale assessing the symptoms of psychosis should assess delusions, hallucinations, formal thought disorders, motor disturbances and cognitive disturbances. Convergent validity assesses how much test items agree with the findings of an alternative procedure thought to measure the same construct.

Incremental validity refers to the extent to which a new instrument is superior to an existing one in measuring what it is intended to measure. Predictive validity helps in predicting a particular aspect of future health status.

13. E The values continue up to infinity.

A normal or gaussian distribution has a number of properties: it is a bell-shaped curve, it is a unimodal symmetrical curve about the mean, i.e. if a line is drawn at the centre of the distribution each side forms the mirror image of the other, and it extends indefinitely to the right and left. The tails of the curve never touch the horizontal axis of the graph and continue to infinity.

The mean, median and mode are equal. It is a good approximation for many naturally occurring continuous variables such as height, body mass, white blood cell count and different types of experimental errors. There is nothing intrinsically wrong when a continuous distribution does not follow the normal distribution and, hence, some prefer the term 'gaussian distribution'.

14. C 3

Standard error is a measure of uncertainty or dispersion of a point estimate, e.g. the sample mean. It is used to construct confidence intervals. The standard error of the mean is the standard deviation (SD) of the sampling distribution of $\bar{x}$. The SD is the square root of the variance, and is a measure of dispersion in the normal distribution. In this question, SD = 9, i.e. square root of 81 ($\sqrt{81}$). The standard error of the mean = $SD/\sqrt{N}$ = 9/3 = 3.

When a mean value is calculated for a smaller sample, the mean obtained may not be the actual mean of the total population if the sample size is sufficiently large. The standard error helps to understand this difference. The larger the sample size, the smaller the standard error of the mean, and vice versa.

15. C κ statistics

Cohen's k is a measure of interrater reliability for qualitative (categorical) items. α is used to denote level of significance, and is most appropriate when different categories of measurement are being recorded. It is also the symbol used to denote type 1 error α. β is used to denote type 2 error. Interrater reliability is the agreement or consensus among raters.

16. C Median

In a descriptive data sample, usually the mean is used as a measure of central tendency. However, if the data are skewed then the median is a better descriptor of central tendency. In a normally distributed sample, mean = median = mode. In positively skewed data, mean > median > mode. In negatively skewed data, mean < median < mode. Interquartile range and standard deviation are the measures of spread.

17. A IQ of students in a classroom

Variables can be continuous or discrete. Continuous variables can follow a normal distribution, e.g. height of boys in a class, IQ scores in a population. Discrete variables can be binary or form discrete categories.

18. B 0.24

When a test is used to screen a condition or disorder, there are chances that a patient could have the disorder. Pre-test probability is the probability or chance of a person having a condition or disorder even before the diagnostic test is administered. Post-test probability is the chance of a person having the disorder after the administration of the test. In this situation, the likelihood ratio (LR) of a positive test, LR+ = Sn/(1 − Sp) = 0.8/0.1 = 8, where Sn is sensitivity and Sp specificity.

Pre-test odds = Prevalence/(1 − Prevalence) = 0.04/(1 − 0.04) = 0.04

Post-test odds = LR+ × Pre-test odds = 8 × 0.04 = 0.32

Post-test probability = Post-test odds/(1 + Post-test odds) = 0.32/1.32 = 0.24.

19. A A test that perfectly discriminates between the two groups would yield a 'curve' that coincided with the left and top sides of the plot.

The ROC curve is useful in evaluating the diagnostic accuracy of a test. The curve is obtained by plotting sensitivity on the y axis and 1 − specificity on the x axis. If the diagnostic accuracy of a test is very low, a straight line will be formed that runs across the graph. A test that has good diagnostic accuracy would yield a curve, which helps to calculate a reasonable cut-off value.

20. C −1 to +1

This is a measure of correlation between two or more variables. The numerical value of the coefficient of correlation represents the degree of correlation between the variables. Correlation coefficient values range from −1 to +1. A correlation coefficient of −1 means a negative correlation and a value of +1 means a positive correlation. Most values lie between these.

21. B Cronbach's α coefficient

In this study, two parts of a scale were assessed against each other for internal consistency. It is measured using Cronbach's α coefficient. Cohen's κ is used to assess internal consistency. The rest of the answers are distractors. Wilks' λ distribution is used in multivariate hypothesis testing, especially with regard to the likelihood ratio test and multivariate analysis.

22. D The null hypothesis states that there is no difference between two populations.

In hypothesis testing, the null hypothesis is tested directly. The alternative hypothesis is a statement that formalises research questions. The null hypothesis nullifies it. As the null hypothesis states that there is no difference between populations of study, there is no direction of difference. The alternative hypothesis could be expressed with direction of difference. Both the null and the alternative hypotheses are statements about populations and do not refer to samples or a particular number of sets. Even when two samples are selected from the same population, it is highly unlikely that the two sample means will be exactly the same. When samples are randomly selected from the same population, any observed difference between them is due to random variation.

23. A Confounder

This is a variable that affects both dependent and independent variables without direct involvement in the causal pathway. A confounder is in fact an independent risk or protective factor for a disease that changes its course due to another exposure. It can lead to a false association, i.e. positive confounding, or a true association, i.e. negative confounding. A variable is defined as an attribute or quantity that varies from one participant to another. An independent variable is the variable that is modified by a researcher to test a dependent variable. A dependent variable is 'dependent' on the independent variable. The variable that affects the outcome or a dependent variable is called the effect modifier. A random variable may be construed as a numerical quantity, the observed value of which is defined by a chance mechanism. In the given study, anticholinergic drugs can reduce the absorption of antipsychotics, and may also affect the extrapyramidal side effects.

24. B The lower the level of significance, the lower the probability of rejecting the null hypothesis.

A type 1 error is denoted by the letter α and a type 2 error by the letter β. A type 1 error is the probability of rejecting a true or correct null hypothesis. A type 2 error is the probability of accepting a null hypothesis when it is not true. The higher the level of significance, the higher the probability of the rejecting null hypothesis and the higher the probability of making a type 1 error. The lower the level of significance, the lower the probability of rejecting the null hypothesis and the lower the probability of making a type 1 error.

25. B The correlation coefficient can be used to express the association.

If the outcome is measured as continuous, regression methods and correlation coefficients are used to express the association. In this question, the outcome is measured as a continuum of psychotic symptoms. If the outcome were measured as categorical values such as presence or absence of psychosis, proportions or percentages could be used. An association helps us to find whether a particular factor is associated with the outcome. It doesn't tell us about causative factors. When a group exposed to a particular factor is associated with fewer chances of an outcome, that factor is a protective factor.

26. C 0.008

The absolute excess risk is also known as the attributable risk (AR) or risk difference.

AR = Incidence (exposed) − Incidence (non-exposed),

i.e. 10/1000 − 2/1000 = 8/1000

= 0.008.

27. C 5

The relative risk (RR) is the incidence among exposed individuals divided by the incidence among non-exposed individuals:

RR = 0.01/0.002 = 5.

If the incidence among non-exposed individuals is very small, the RR may be large but still not important. In these situations, the attributable risk is more informative. When we use the attributable risk, information is not lost. Unemployment and low socioeconomic status could be the results of schizophrenia, i.e. reverse causality. If the absolute risk is 0, the factor under investigation makes no difference. If the RR is 1, the factor under investigation also makes no difference.

28. A 0.0012

Population attributable risk (PAR) = Prevalence × AR = 0.15 × 0.008 = 0.0012.

The PAR helps us to calculate the impact of a risk factor at the population level. If a large number of the population is at negligible risk, the impact of the risk for that group is diluted and becomes less important at the population level.

29. C Roughly 68% of all scores lie within 1 SD on either side of the mean score.

For data that are normally distributed, the SD conveys very useful information about the spread of the data. About two-thirds of the data (68.2%) lie within 1 SD on either side of the mean score, and about 95% of the scores lie within 2 SDs on either side of the mean score.

30. A ANOVA

This is a parametric test; the rest are non-parametric tests. ANOVA is used to compare three or more groups on a single continuous measure. It tests the null hypothesis that the mean values of three or more groups are equal. There are different types of ANOVA: one way between groups, one-way repeated measures, two way between groups, two-way repeated measures, and multivariate analysis of variance, which is based on a general linear model. ANOVA is also available for non-parametric data. The Kruskal–Wallis test (one independent grouping only) is a non-parametric equivalent of ANOVA. The Whitney–Mann–Wilcoxon test is distribution free and based on ranked values. It is useful to compare the medians of two independent groups. Friedman's test is a non-parametric test and it is useful in detecting differences in treatments across various attempts. Wilcoxon's signed rank test is a non-parametric and distribution-free test for measuring the difference between two paired samples.

31. D The tail of *t* distribution inflate inversely in relation to the sample number.

The Student's *t*-test is a parametric test used to compare the means of two samples or treatments. It compares the difference between two means in relation to the variation in the data. It is expressed as the standard deviation of the difference between the means. The *z*-test and the Student's *t*-test are parametric tests. The *z*-test is a hypothesis-testing technique; the sample should be normally distributed. It is not routinely used. To apply the Student's *t*-test, the observations must be independent. The Student's *t*-test is commonly used. The *t* distributions are not same as normal distributions: the tail of the *t* distribution is inversely related to the sample number. If the sample number is small, then the tails are more inflated. If the sample number is infinite, then the tails are thin and the *t* and *z* values will be same. In this case, *t* distribution is identical to normal distribution.

32. C Publication bias

A funnel plot is used to evaluate the presence of publication bias in a systematic review or a meta-analysis. It is a plot of the study effect size against its precision. The effect size is measured as a mean difference or standardised difference for continuous data. For dichotomous data or event-like data, the relative risk or odds ratio is calculated. Input of all the studies produces the graph. If the studies are free of bias, a funnel-shaped plot is formed. Otherwise the curve will not have a uniform spread of studies.

33. D The last observation carried forward could be used to correct the error due to loss of follow-up.

Even though 55 patients improved out of the 60 patients who remained in the study, we cannot say that the drug 'Safe' is more effective than imipramine. Patients could drop out of a trial for many reasons. Some could have actually improved as a result of the natural course of the illness and dropped out. Some patients could have dropped out because of the side effects. The bias that arises due to loss of follow-up is called 'attrition bias'. There are methods to account for patients who drop out of studies, e.g. last observation carried forward (LOCF) and worst-case scenario. In LOCF, the scores on the last assessment before the drop-out are removed and carried over to the end of the study. However, the LOCF has limitations for both clinical and statistical reasons. Patients dropping out for reasons other than treatment failure might be regarded as treatment failure. LOCF may over- or underestimate the benefits of treatment depending on the condition and treatment investigated. Per protocol analysis includes only patients who completed the course of treatment, so they may not give the true picture.

34. A Construct validity

This refers to the extent to which a test measures a condition. It is done by various methods. Two commonly used methods are: (1) factor analysis and (2) discriminant analysis. Face validity is assessing the 'face value' of the test. It is done by asking the opinion of experts in the area, as well as from people who use it, e.g. getting feedback from trainees and examiners after the RCPsych exam results. Content validity refers to the extent to which a questionnaire is representative of all the relevant items that could have been chosen, e.g. a questionnaire on depression could have high content validity if it covered all the domains such as biological symptoms, cognitive symptoms, negative cognitions and psychological symptoms.

Criterion validity is divided into concurrent validity and predictive validity. Concurrent validity measures the level of agreement between a test and the gold standard in that area. Predictive validity refers to how much a test can predict future health status.

Answers: MCQs

35. E Random error

In scientific experiments, many types of errors can occur. Errors distort the results of a study. When an error is non-systematic, it is called a random error.

A random error is unpredictable and closely related to the study's precision. If there is a systematic error that results in distortion of the results, it is called a bias. Omission can result in distorted results.

36. C 0.54

Coefficient of non-determination = 1 − Coefficient of determination

Coefficient of determination = Correlation coefficient^2, i.e. $0.68 \times 0.68 = 0.46$.

Therefore:

Coefficient of non-determination = 0.54.

The coefficient of determination helps us to find information about proportions and predictability, e.g. if the coefficient of determination is very high, it tells us that total variability in one variable is predicated using the relationship between two variables. On the other hand, if the coefficient of non-determination is high this tells us that the variability in one variable is not explained by the relationship between the two variables.

37. C Cost-effectiveness analysis

Different types of economic evaluations are used in research studies. If an evaluation is used to assess the choice between two alternative treatments for the same patient group, a cost-effectiveness analysis is used. In this analysis, costs are related to a clinical output measure such as life-years gained or another generic outcome measure. This allows comparisons of 'relative (productive) efficiency', so maximising a health outcome for a given cost per outcome. However, cost-effectiveness analysis cannot compare different outcomes or even choose between interventions providing more benefit at greater cost or less benefit at lower cost. When both health and non-health effects are measured after an intervention, a cost–consequence analysis may be useful. A cost–benefit analysis is an economic analysis and it compares the costs and outcomes of two or more therapeutic interventions in terms of monetary value.

38. C Incremental cost-effectiveness ratio

The primary outcome of a cost–utility analysis is the incremental cost-effectiveness ratio (ICER). This is the ratio of the change in costs to incremental benefits of a therapeutic treatment or intervention. ICER is an equation that provides practical guidance to make decisions about healthcare interventions. It is also known as cost per quality-adjusted life-year (QALY).

$ICER = (C1 - C2)/(E1 - E2)$,

where C1 = cost of intervention group, C2 = cost of control group, E1 = effect in intervention group and E2 = effect in control group.

If a treatment is more effective at the same or less cost than an alternative, the interpretation is simple. When a more expensive and more effective treatment is compared with an existing treatment, interpretation of the data is less straightforward. In this situation, the term 'incremental cost' is used, which refers to the additional cost per unit of healthcare gain by switching from less to more expensive treatment. Cost–benefit analysis measures all the inputs and outputs in monetary terms, e.g. costs of drugs, investigations and staff against costs of time off work with and without treatment. Cost–utility analysis measures an output such as the QALY and combines quantitative and qualitative information of the amount of life gained and the relative quality of that to the individual.

39. C 0.71

Sensitivity of a test is also called the true positive rate of the test. It is the proportion of cases identified by the test, i.e. the probability of a positive test in individuals who have the disease (**Table 2.3**).

Table 2.3 A 2 × 2 table

Personality disorder questionnaire	Structured interview by psychologist		Total
	Personality disorder diagnosed	Personality disorder not diagnosed	
Personality disorder diagnosed	50 (a)	110 (b)	160 (a + c)
Personality disorder not diagnosed	20 (c)	820 (d)	840 (c + d)
Total	70 (a + c)	930 (b + d)	1000 total

Formula for calculating sensitivity is:
Sensitivity (Sn) = $a/(a + c)$ = 50/70 = 0.71.

40. D 0.88

The specificity of a test is also called a true negative rate. It is the probability of a negative test in individuals who do not have a disease, i.e. proportion of non-cases identified by the test:

Specificity (Sp) = $d/(b + d)$ = 820/930 = 0.88.

41. A 0.31

The positive predictive value (PPV) is the probability of a participant with a positive test having a target disease, i.e. the proportion of individuals who have a positive test result who have the disease. It is also known as a posterior probability of the disorder or a post-test probability of the disorder for a positive test.

PPV = $a/(a + b)$ = 50/160 = 0.31.

42. E 0.97

The negative predictive value (NPV) is the probability of a participant with a negative test not having a target disease, i.e. the proportion of individuals who have a negative test result who do not have the disease. It is also known as a posterior probability of the disorder or a post-test probability of the disorder for a negative test.

NPV = $d/(c + d)$ = 820/840 = 0.97.

43. E 5.91

The likelihood ratio for a positive test result (LR+) tells us the likelihood that a positive test result comes from an individual who is affected by the disease rather than from an individual who does not have a disease:

LR+ = Sensitivity/(1 − Specificity) = 0.71/(1 − 0.88) = 5.91.

Answers: MCQs

44. A 0.32

The likelihood ratio for a negative test result (LR-) tells us the likelihood that a negative test result comes from an individual who is affected by the disease rather than from an individual who does not have a disease:

LR- = (1 − Sensitivity)/Specificity = (1 − 0.71)/0.88 = 0.32.

45. B 0.07

The prevalence of a disease is the ratio of the number of cases or people affected by the disease in the target population divided by the total number of the population:

Prevalence = Number of people with disease/Total number = 70/1000 = 0.07.

46. C The predictive values of a test setting cannot be generalised to a general population.

The accuracy of a test refers to the proportion of true cases detected by the test, i.e. both positive and negative. Accuracy may be misleading if it is not quoted with other values such as sensitivity and specificity. The importance of accuracy varies with these values, so it is not a very useful indicator of the test on its own.

The predictive values of a test setting cannot be generalised to a general population unless the test is conducted in the same population. The predictive values of a test depend on the prevalence of disease in the population of interest. Independent prevalence rates of the population are needed to understand predictive values in the context of the population.

Sensitivity and specificity of the test can be generalised to the general population.

47. C It is calculated by using the ranks of data observations.

Spearman's correlation coefficient examines data that are not normal in distribution, or when the data being considered are ordinal or discrete. All the rest are applicable to Pearson's correlation coefficient between two normally distributed continuous variables.

48. A When it is desirable to compare an intervention for this condition with an intervention for a different condition.

Cost–benefit analysis converts all the costs and consequences of a clinical intervention into the same units, usually monetary. Different interventions can be compared, even when the outcomes are very different.

49. B 2.67

The odds of improvement are 40/10 and 30/20, respectively. The odds ratio (OR) for improving is 40/10 divided by 30/20, which is 2.67.

50. D It is the most commonly used adaptive method of randomisation.

Minimisation is the most commonly used adaptive method of randomisation. It involves identifying a few important prognostic factors in a trial and then applying the weighting system. Every subsequent participant is then randomised to the treatment group that would cause the least imbalance to the overall distribution of weighted prognostic factors among the compared groups. Minimisation is performed to ensure an overall balance in the distribution of the more important prognostic factors among the trial's various treatment groups.

51. B Observational methods allow qualitative researchers to assess human behaviours and interactions first hand, along with the impact that these behaviours may have on the subject of interest.

Observational methods are best suited for qualitative (not quantitative) research questions that are loaded with behavioural or procedural issues. The major limitation of the observation method is that the very presence of an observer can alter people's behaviour. Qualitative researchers must embark on justifiable covert observational methods to overcome this problem.

Observational methods (covert and overt) are frequently used in the area of health management to identify areas of weakness and possible strategies for healthcare management.

52. D Simple correlations are a satisfactory measure of reliability of a scale, whether these are calculated as the correlation between two halves or the average of all the correlations among the items.

Intrarater reliability is the extent to which one rater is stable over time. Content or sampling validity (not reliability) is the completeness of assessment of the phenomenon. Split-half scale reliability is the comparison between two halves of a scale. Reliability can be quantified as a correlation coefficient.

53. B Direct contact surveys include self-completed questionnaires, either situational or surveys of records.

Surveys are the systematic collection of information. The term 'survey' is more accurately applicable to two-phase epidemiological surveys, i.e. a screening questionnaire followed by an interview. They are generally cross-sectional studies of incidence and prevalence. To establish the incidence and prevalence of a disorder, it is not necessary to have a control group. If the surveys are carried out on two separate occasions, the incidence and predictors of a disorder may be studied. These help to identify associations of a disorder by comparing the rates in different areas or the associations in participants with and without the disorder. Surveys involving no contact with responders include self-completed questionnaires and surveys of records. They can helpfully inform health service planning.

54. B The median survival time is usually presented using p values and confidence intervals.

The median survival time is defined as the duration from the start of a study that coincides with a 0.5 probability of survival. In terms of clinical relevance, the median survival time is estimated as the smallest survival time for which the survivor function is considered ≤0.5. It refers to how long patients survive with a disease in general or after a specific treatment. It means that half the patients are expected to be alive after the diagnosis, and the probability of survival beyond that time is approximately 50%. The confidence interval of the median survival time is calculated by using a robust non-parametric method. The median survival time cannot be estimated for as long as survival times remain >0.5. It is useful in estimating survival and prognosis of a group of patients with serious conditions. Survival times are generally not felt to obey a normal distribution. The mean survival time is estimated as the area under the survival curve. It is recommended that the entire range of data be used to determine the estimator. The area under the estimate of the Kaplan–Meier survival curve is the non-parametric estimate of the mean survival time.

55. B Hawthorne's effect

This phenomenon occurs because just the mere clinical contact in a study can have a positive 'feel-good' effect in the way that study participants perceive their symptoms. Needless to say, this effect can produce artificially encouraging data on the beneficial effects of experimental and control treatments. To counteract Hawthorne's effect, a third silent group may be created in addition to experimental and control groups. This third group would usually have no further contact with the trial after the recruitment phase. The results of the silent groups can then be compared to assess for Hawthorne's effect at the end of the trial. The placebo effect refers to the non-therapeutic effects of the inactive intervention. It can occur with any intervention given or taken with sufficient interest and enthusiasm. Random effect analyses are used when heterogeneity is present. They do not assume a single underlying treatment effect but assume an average treatment effect across various studies. Vicarious or observational learning occurs through observing the behaviour of other people.

56. A Cross-over trial

In these trials, all participants receive two or more interventions in succession. The participants may be randomised to receive a particular intervention, first or second. These trials are a real option to study relatively rare diseases where the small numbers of participants may not allow a randomised, parallel, group-controlled trial. They also allow for overcoming any participant's ethical dilemma about not receiving an active intervention. The participants act as their own controls. However, there are several disadvantages: uncertainty about the duration of the trial to ensure therapeutic effects, fluctuations in disease condition and carry-over effects.

57. D It gives a low percentage of false-negative results.

When a test suggests infection (or whatever it is detecting) in an unaffected individual, it is referred to as a false positive. A high specificity test will give a low percentage of false positives. When a test is negative in a patient who in fact has the infection, it is called a false-negative test. Highly sensitive tests will give a low percentage of false negatives.

58. C Programmes not targeting depression can lead to a reduction in the symptoms of depression.

Social support programmes had a lower effect size, except in older people where they performed better. Multimodal programmes with at least three methods were significantly better. Behavioural programmes had the lowest effect size, whereas competence enhancement programmes had the largest effect size.

59. C Bipolar III

There has been the recent emergence of bipolar spectrum based on clinical, epidemiological, familial and genetic lines. Bipolar III disorder has been described as the mood disorder in which a patient can present with recurrent depressive episodes. Treatment with antidepressants could lead to hypomanic episodes. Bipolar I disorder is the well-described mood disorder characterised by episodes of mania and depression. Bipolar II disorder is characterised by depressive episodes and hypomanic episodes (may not be antidepressant induced).

60. A 5–10%

The association of epilepsy with psychosis is well researched but still not clearly understood. However, the well-known entity schizophrenia-like psychosis of epilepsy (SLPE) is commonly seen in patients with temporal lobe epilepsy. It is a form of post-ictal psychosis usually seen after 10–15 years of epileptic illness. There is no clear correlation with the severity of the epilepsy and prevalence of the psychosis. The prevalence of psychosis in temporal lobe epilepsy is 5–10% – against the 1% prevalence of psychosis in the general population.

61. D Serotonin–noradrenaline reuptake inhibitors

Antidepressants may lower the seizure threshold in individuals who are prone to them. Hence in patients with epilepsy the choice of antidepressants is limited. SSRIs are generally considered safe in patients with epilepsy and the SNRIs (serotonin–noradrenaline reuptake inhibitors) are also considered safe.

62. A Compliance with treatment

Psychiatric morbidities will affect the course and prognosis of HIV/AIDS by several mechanisms, including the function of immunity, compliance of HIV/AIDS patient with treatment and involvement in risk behaviours.

63. C Cocaine

Table 2.4 describes the possible effects of drugs used in pregnancy.

Table 2.4 Effects of drugs in pregnancy	
Drug	Fetal and neonatal effects
Amphetamines	Miscarriage, IUGR, premature delivery
Cannabis	Possible dose-related IUGR, premature delivery
Cocaine	Intracranial haemorrhage, IUGR, abruption placenta, SIDS, premature delivery
Methadone	IUGR, decreased head circumference, raised PMR, SIDS
Nicotine	Miscarriage, IUGR, premature delivery
IUGR, intrauterine growth retardation; PMR, perinatal mortality rate; SIDS, sudden infant death syndrome.	

64. C Selective serotonin reuptake inhibitors

In this scenario, the condition is characterised by uncontrollable laughing, crying or both, which are exaggerated or completely out of context. It occurs in patients with neurological disorders such as traumatic brain injury (5–11% in year 1), multiple sclerosis (10%), amyotrophic lateral sclerosis (49%), stroke (11–34%) and Parkinson's disease (5%). The first line of treatment is a selective serotonin reuptake inhibitor (SSRI) medication. If the patient is unable to tolerate this or has significant side effects, drugs such as tricyclic antidepressants (TCAs), quinidine plus dextromethorphan and dopaminergic drugs can be used.

Answers: MCQs

65. B Degree to which the treating dose exceeds the seizure threshold

The extent to which the treatment dose exceeds the seizure threshold correlates directly with the efficacy of the treatment. For unilateral ECT, an effective treatment dose can be between 2.5 and 6 times the seizure threshold and, in bilateral ECT, it can be 1.5–2 times the seizure threshold. Such a dose results in a generalised symmetrical cerebral seizure activity of sufficient duration.

66. A Geographical separation may be necessary to reduce risks.

Morbid jealousy is a symptom rather than a diagnosis and it is otherwise known as Othello's syndrome. It is usually associated with alcohol and substance misuse. Depression, schizophrenia, organic brain disease and sexual dysfunction are also known associations. Morbid jealousy is a disorder of thought content and can take the form of a delusion, obsession and overvalued ideas in various combinations. Treatment involves identification of the underlying cause and appropriate treatment. Occasionally, geographical separation may be the only solution.

67. C It is associated with a low self-esteem.

Morbid jealousy is mostly seen in males. Evidence-seeking behaviour increases the risks of arguments and violence. Most homicides by sufferers are of the current or ex-partner and about 5–7% of homicides are of the suspected rivals. Low self-esteem, sexual dysfunction and substance misuse are the known classic associations.

68. E Explanation, reassurance and support by a health visitor

Postpartum mental health problems range from maternity blues to puerperal psychosis. This woman has maternity blues, which is seen in between half and two-thirds of women after a normal delivery. Symptoms reach their peak on day 3 or 4 postpartum. Sleep problems are to be expected anyway with a new baby. Postnatal depression occurs in around 10% of women in the early weeks of the postpartum period and will be similar to a depressive episode. The condition responds to supportive and practical non-pharmacological treatments or antidepressants, or the woman may need referral to a specialist service. Postpartum psychosis needs admission but is unlikely in this case.

69. B Epilepsy

Electroconvulsive therapy (ECT) is a useful treatment option for patients with severe depression refractory to medication or those with psychotic symptoms. Important side effects include headache, nausea, short-term memory impairment – both anterograde and retrograde – cardiac arrhythmias, musculoskeletal problems such as muscle soreness, shoulder dislocations, etc. ECT itself has an antiepileptic effect and increases the threshold for seizures. Therefore, the dose of electric charge needs to be increased with every ECT treatment.

70. B Depression

This patient appears to have Parkinson's disease – a classic triad of features: bradykinesia, tremor and rigidity. Gait problems (festinating gait) are very common. There could also be postural instability, which can present as frequent falls. The most common psychiatric problem is depression, with 40% of patients with Parkinson's disease developing depression during the course of their illness. Dementia is less common than depression. Psychosis can also occur but is not as common. The dopaminergic drugs used to treat Parkinson's disease can also contribute to cause psychotic or mood symptoms.

71. D RD Laing

These views were expressed by RD Laing, who was one of the most influential people in the anti-psychiatry movement, along with Szaz, Foucault and Cooper. Anti-psychiatry is a configuration of groups and theoretical constructs that emerged in the 1960s, and questioned the fundamental assumptions and practices of psychiatry. Thomas Szaz wrote Myth of Mental Illness. Goffman's main contribution to psychiatry was his work on institutionalisation of psychiatric patients. Foucault wrote Madness and Civilization: A history of insanity in the age of reason.

72. E SOFAS (Social and Occupational Functioning Assessment Scale)

This can be used to track a patient's progress in social and occupational areas, regardless of psychiatric diagnosis and the severity of the patient's psychological symptoms. It rates functioning on a continuum from 1 to 100.

73. C CIWA (Clinical Institute Withdrawal Assessment)

This is used to assess the withdrawal symptoms during detoxification, and is clinician rated. The withdrawal signs are scored and a score >15 is associated with increased risk of withdrawal seizures or delirium tremens. CAGE, AUDIT and MAST are used in primary care for the screening of alcohol dependence and DAST is used in substance misuse disorders as a screening tool.

74. C Left frontal stroke lesions

These lesions are a high risk factor for depression. Worsening of depressive symptoms is associated with subcortical white matter lesions. Persistent symptoms over 2 consecutive years are due to small lesions in basal ganglia or large cerebral cortical lesions.

75. D There is a higher incidence of elevated thyroid antibodies.

Moya-moya is a progressive occlusive disease of the cerebral vasculature (usually bilateral), especially the circle of Willis and the arteries that feed it. There is intimal thickening of the walls of the end-portions of the internal carotid vessels. In Japanese moya-moya does mean 'puff of smoke'. Occlusion of the main vessels causes a network of abnormal small collateral vessels, which when seen on angiography appear as a puff of smoke. There is a familial form (about 15% of patients), autosomal dominant with incomplete penetrance; it depends on age and genomic imprinting factors. There is a higher incidence of elevated thyroid antibodies. Cerebral ischaemic events are common in children and haemorrhagic events in adults.

76. E The psychosis is usually of a paranoid type with a richness of affective symptoms.

About 2–9% of patients with epilepsy have psychotic disorders, and about half of patients with epilepsy and psychosis could be diagnosed with schizophrenia. Psychoses closely linked to seizures

77. B Antisocial behaviour before the head injury

This is a major predictor of aggression after a head injury. Other predictors are personality change with disinhibition or impulsivity, epilepsy, AEDs, and confusion and disorientation. If aggression emerges, either during confusion or shortly after its resolution, it suggests the likelihood of an organic pathology. If the aggression has a pattern of being highly stereotyped, erupts over seconds with no or trivial triggers, is bizarre and against a background of calm behaviour, then it suggests the possibility of epilepsy.

78. B Cerebral atrophy is in the dorsofrontal regions.

Alcohol-related dementia accounts for 10% of cases in the dementia population. Cerebral atrophy in the dorsofrontal regions contributes to 20–25% of cognitive impairment in mid-adulthood. The earlier the onset, the poorer the prognosis, and the prevalence is high in socioeconomically deprived areas.

79. A Early behavioural symptoms include apathy, reduced spontaneity and emotional responsivity.

HIV-associated dementia that is usually insidious in onset presents with early cognitive symptoms and early behavioural symptoms (there is reduced emotional responsivity and spontaneity, apathy and social withdrawal). There is early mental slowing, loss of concentration and forgetfulness, and the performance of complex mental sequential tasks is affected. Loss of balance, incoordination, weakness of legs and clumsiness occur early in the course of the disease. Ocular motility tests are abnormal and there is saccadic inaccuracy or slowing. Depression, psychotic symptoms and emotional lability with irritability may also occur. As the disease progresses, there is linguistic difficulties with word finding, eventually progressing to mutism in the late stages.

80. E The onset is usually in the 45- to 75-year age group

CJD is characterised by rapidly progressive dementia, speech difficulties, jerky movements, ataxia, rigid posture and seizures. The peak age of onset is 60–65. About 10% of cases of CJD present initially with cerebellar ataxia and 70% die within 6 months. Within weeks of the onset, the patient progresses to akinetic mutism. All routine blood investigations (except raised serum transaminases or alkaline phosphatase), along with immunological markers and acute phase proteins, are within normal limits. There is a build-up of the abnormal prion protein, leading to the formation of amyloids.

81. C Combination of lamotrigine and antidepressant drug

Depersonalisation syndrome is characterised by persistent or recurrent feelings of being detached from one's own mental processes or body. It is thought to be caused by severe traumatic life experiences such as childhood abuse, accidents, torture, war and bad drug trips. Primary depersonalisation syndrome is mostly resistant to treatment. Clinical trials that combine an antipsychotic and clomipramine did not show any evidence of improvement in primary depersonalisation disorder. Opioid antagonists have shown transient symptom reduction with naloxone infusion and some efficacy with oral naltrexone. The lamotrigine and antidepressant combination has been found to be the most useful in depersonalisation syndrome. Cognitive–behaviour therapy, trancranial magnetic stimulation and modafinil have a role in the treatment of this disorder.

82. D The outcome for anorexic men is remarkably similar to that for women.

The frequency of anorexia nervosa is less among men. Poor prognosis in anorexic men is associated with the absence of normal adolescent sexual behaviour, a long duration of illness, severe weight loss and premorbid fantasy. Testicular function is disturbed when the patient is emaciated. A good outcome predictor in anorexic men is previous sexual activity whereas a disturbed relationship with a parent in childhood leads to a poor prognosis. Overall, the outcome of anorexia nervosa is remarkably similar to that in women. Atypical gender role behaviour does not increase the risk of anorexia nervosa in men. A quarter of anorexic men tend to have homosexual tendencies.

83. D Premature ejaculation

The most common sexual problem in men with social phobia is premature ejaculation. SSRIs mainly affect the triggering of orgasm, thus causing delayed ejaculation. Men with low sexual desire also report a reduction of 'spontaneous' erections. Premature ejaculation can be primary or secondary. Secondary premature ejaculation is usually confounded by problems with erection. Premature ejaculation can be further divided into global premature ejaculation, which occurs with all sexual partners, and situational premature ejaculation, which occurs in certain situations or with particular partners. SSRIs such as paroxetine (short acting), fluoxetine and sertraline, clomipramine and tramadol are useful in premature ejaculation.

84. C Paranoid personality disorder

This is found in 0.5–1% of the general population and 10–20% of psychiatric patients. It has a hereditary relationship with schizophrenia and delusional disorder. Pathological jealousy is a common presentation in paranoid personality disorder. Those with avoidant personality disorder are preoccupied with their own shortcomings and avoid social interactions because they fear being rejected, ridiculed or humiliated. They will form relationships with others only when they believe that they will not be rejected. Those with narcissistic personality disorder are excessively preoccupied with self-importance, power, prestige and vanity. It involves arrogant behaviour and lack of empathy for others. Those with schizotypal personality disorder are characterised by being anxious in social situations, needing social isolation, and having odd behaviour, odd thinking and unconventional beliefs, e.g. telepathy. These people are described as odd and eccentric, and usually have few if any close relationships.

85. C Grandiosity

Although both personality disorders are strikingly similar, phenomenologically grandiosity is the best discriminator present in narcissistic personality disorder. In this disorder, there is better impulse control, greater social adjustment, better anxiety tolerance, a lesser danger of regressive fragmentation, fewer suicide attempts and fewer psychotic episodes. Borderline personality disorder is characterised by intense and unstable interpersonal relationships, impulsive behaviour, unusual variability and depth of moods, unstable self-image and sense of self, feeling of abandonment, self-harm and suicidal behaviour.

86. A Assessment of vitamin levels

This is a case of a chronic deficiency of niacin (vitamin B_3) or tryptophan, which causes pellagra, and is the result of poor dietary intake. Vitamin B_3 is one of the eight B-complex vitamins. It plays an important role in the metabolism of proteins and carbohydrates, blood circulation and the functioning of the nervous system. It is involved in the synthesis of various hormones such as insulin, sex hormones, cortisone and thyroxine. Vitamin B_3 deficiency causes forgetfulness, irritability, insomnia, nervousness and pellagra, which is characterised by bilateral dermatitis (stocking and glove), diarrhoea and dementia. Severe and prolonged vitamin B_3 deficiency may cause depression and neurasthenia. Investigation of urea and electrolytes may help but not explain dermatitis and memory problems. MRI will not explain dermatitis or diarrhoea but may throw some light on the structure of the brain. Skin biopsy will help only with skin lesions. Stool examination will not explain the other symptoms.

87. C Liver biopsy

This patient probably has Wilson's disease. Liver biopsy is the most diagnostic definitive test. Progressive hepatolenticular degeneration, or Wilson's disease, is a genetic disorder of copper metabolism, and is an autosomal recessive disorder. In Wilson's disease, there is a copper overload in the liver, which leads to accumulation of copper in the tissues. It is characterised by psychiatric symptoms (e.g. depression, anxiety and psychosis) and neurological symptoms (e.g. parkinsonism, ataxia, choreoathetoid movements) at a young age. Kayser–Fleischer rings in the cornea of the eyes are a pathognomonic sign in these patients. Abnormally decreased serum ceruloplasmin and increased copper levels in the urine usually confirm the diagnosis. However, liver biopsy is the most definitive investigation. Copper works as a cofactor for a number of enzymes such as ceruloplasmin, cytochrome c oxidase, dopamine β-hydroxylase, superoxide dismutase and tyrosinase.

88. C Decreased serum ceruloplasmin and increased copper in urine

Wilson's disease manifests as neurological and psychiatric symptoms and liver disease. About half the people with Wilson's disease have neurological (e.g. parkinsonism, ataxia, choreoathetoid movements) or psychiatric problems (e.g. depression, anxiety and psychosis). Kayser–Fleischer rings are visible around the iris on slit-lamp examination. Decreased serum ceruloplasmin and increased copper in the urine confirm the diagnosis.

89. B In psychiatric wards, delirium tremens is probably the most common form of delirium seen.

Children are more susceptible to delirium than adults and may develop delirium with any severe acute illness, most commonly pyrexia due to an acute infection. Elderly people are considerably more susceptible than younger adults. Prescription of multiple medicines (including psychotropics, especially hypnotics), dehydration and chronic medical conditions are frequently contributing factors. Those with pre-existing dementia are especially vulnerable to developing delirium; indeed, an episode of delirium is frequently the reason for first presentation to medical services among patients with dementia. Delirium occurs in about 15% of all general medical and surgical inpatients. In adult psychiatry, delirium tremens is probably the most common form of delirium seen.

90. D Tau

Neurofibrillary tangles are found in the pathogenesis of Alzheimer's disease. They are made up of hyperphosphorylated tau proteins. Amyloid plaques are another finding in the pathogenesis of Alzheimer's disease.

91. D Posterior parietal cortex sparing

A SPECT (single-photon computed tomography) scan using ^{99m}Tc-labelled HMPAO (hexamethylpropylene amine oxime) (for the blood flow) shows global reduction, especially in the posterior parietotemporal region in Alzheimer's disease. A variable pattern is seen in vascular dementia, depending on the location of infarcts. There is global reduction, especially in occipital region and relatively unaffected temporal lobes in dementia with Lewy bodies.

92. A Circadian rhythm sleep disorders

EEG features in circadian rhythm sleep disorders (irregular sleep–wake pattern) include reduced sleep spindles and K-complexes. Changes associated with and underlying cerebral condition may also be present.

Other sleep disorders related to EEG changes include:

- Idiopathic insomnia/childhood-onset insomnia: varied, minor, non-specific abnormalities
- Narcolepsy: features of drowsiness; eye opening may increase α activity
- Recurrent hypersomnia/Kleine–Levin syndrome: low-voltage slow activity or diffuse α activity
- Non-24-hour sleep–wake syndrome: changes as for circadian rhythm sleep disorders
- Confusional arousals/sleep drunkenness: slow activity during episodes
- Sleep paralysis: slow activity and/or pendular eye movements during episode
- Sleep enuresis: occasionally associated with epilepsy, so discharges may be found.

93. D They understand that death involves permanent separation.

The child's ability to comprehend various components of the concept of death has been well studied. The consensus is that:

- By 5 years of age, most children of normal intelligence can understand that death leads to a state where a person is immobile and cannot sense or feel anything. They also develop the concept that death is irreversible. However, they might not be in a position to give details surrounding bereavement.
- The concept of corporeal deterioration is more difficult for young children to comprehend and is not fully formed until nearer puberty.

94. C Tics can be voluntarily suppressed by the sufferers.

Tic disorders are complex neurodevelopmental disorders that may be diagnosed in psychiatric, paediatric or neurology clinics. A tic is an involuntary, rapid, recurrent, non-rhythmic motor movement or vocal production that is of sudden onset and serves no specific purpose. Tics may be voluntarily suppressed, but sufferers often report that after a period of suppression the tic frequency increases. Tics can also be reproduced voluntarily.

Between 10 and 4% of children will manifest tics at some point during development but most are simple and transient. Gilles de la Tourette's syndrome has a lifetime prevalence of 0.01–1.6%. The male:female ratio is approximately 2:1. The average age of onset is 7 years (range 2–15).

Most children's tics will be transient, disappearing spontaneously after a few weeks or months. Some, however, will show a downward progression.

95. D The Children's Act should be considered under circumstances where parents also refuse treatment.

NICE guidance recommends the following in children with anorexia nervosa who refuse treatment that is deemed essential:

- In children who refuse treatment of anorexia nervosa where there is high risk the treatment should be with the agreement of the person with parental responsibility.
- If the patient as well as the person with parental responsibility refuses treatment then legal advice should be sought and treatment might be initiated using the Mental Health Act or under the Children Act 1989.
- If needed a second opinion from an eating disorder specialist should be sought.

96. D Medication

According to NICE, in children of school age and adolescents with severe ADHD:

- Medication is the first-line treatment.
- Other interventions include educating the parents, group interventions, behavioural and educational interventions.

97. C Most children are troubled by repetitive and intrusive thoughts about the accident.

About one in three (36%) children meets the criteria for PTSD after a range of traumas. Child survivors find it difficult to talk to parents or peers about their trauma to avoid upsetting them. Most children are troubled by repetitive and intrusive thoughts about the accident. Separation difficulties are common in children and also in adolescents. Vivid dissociative flashbacks are uncommon.

98. B Boys have an earlier onset than girls.

About a third of children report that certain triggers initiate their rituals and avoidance of such 'triggers' protects them from OCD symptoms. Boys have an earlier onset than girls. Childhood-onset OCD typically begins late in childhood or early adolescence. Pure obsessions are not common in children. Females report more compulsions and males report more obsessions.

99. E Monozygotic rate of 60–90%

Concordance for autism has been found to be 60–90% in monozygotic twins and between 0 and 10% in dizygotic twins (**Table 2.5**).

Table 2.5 Incidence rates in monozygotic and dizygotic twins

Disorder	Monozygotic concordance rates (%)	Dizygotic concordance rates (%)
ADHD	70–80	30
Anorexia nervosa	55	5
Bulimia nervosa	35	30
Bipolar disorder	60–70	20–30
Depression	40	–
OCD	80–90	50
Gilles de la Tourette's syndrome	50	10
Chronic motor tics	77	30

100. E Make a positive contribution

The five outcomes of 'Every child matters' by the Department of Education include:

1. Be healthy
2. Be safe
3. Enjoy and achieve
4. Make a positive contribution
5. Achieve economic wellbeing.

101. D Section 25 allows the child to be placed in secure accommodation if he or she is likely to abscond.

A child assessment order lasts 7 days and is not for use in emergencies. Both the NSPCC and the local authority can apply for a care order. Anyone can apply for an emergency protection order if concerns are present that a child is in a potentially dangerous environment. Section 25 allows the child to be placed in secure accommodation if he or she is likely to abscond. Wardship has been rendered largely redundant.

102. B 40%

Forward continuity: 40% of children with conduct disorder become delinquent young adults with ongoing behaviour problems and disrupted relationships.

Backward continuity: 90% of young adult delinquents had a conduct disorder as children. A poor outcome is predicted by early onset, a wide range and high total number of symptoms, greater severity and frequency of individual symptoms, pervasiveness across situations (home, school, other) and associated hyperactivity. Parental psychiatric disorder, parental criminality, high hostility and high discord focused on the child also predict poorer outcomes.

103. C Selective mutism

This was formerly known as elective mutism. It is the persistent failure to speak in specific social situations despite speaking appropriately in other settings. The symptoms must last for at least 1 month for a diagnosis to be made. It usually starts before the age of 5 years and is rare (<1%) in the community. It is more common in girls.

104. D Point prevalence of ADHD is about 5%.

The three subtypes of ADHD are: inattentive, hyperactive/impulsive and combined. The most common overlap of symptoms of ADHD is with conduct disorder or oppositional defiant disorder. Stimulants are not contraindicated if co-morbid Giles de la Tourette's syndrome is present, but caution is advised. Medication is more effective than behavioural strategies.

105. D 3–3.5%

Major depressive disorder and bipolar disorder occur with the same frequency in the learning-disabled population as in the general population.

Psychotic disorders, particularly schizophrenia, appear to be more common among learning-disabled individuals. Most studies report a prevalence of 3–3.5% for schizophrenia.

Neurotic disorders were rarely reported in early prevalence literature but recent studies have shown that anxiety disorders, somatoform disorders and dissociative disorders are at least as common in mildly learning-disabled individuals as they are in the general population and are commonly a reason for hospitalisation.

106. A Duchenne muscular dystrophy

Duchenne muscular dystrophy (Xp21.2) is associated with general learning difficulties in 25–30% of cases and occurs only in boys.

Fragile X syndrome (Xq27.3) is associated with general learning difficulties in 50–60% of cases and occurs only in girls.

Klinefelter's syndrome (47,XXY) is not associated with general learning difficulties although the verbal IQ is slightly below average. It occurs in boys only.

Neurofibromatosis (17q11.2) is associated with general learning difficulties in 30–45% of cases and occurs in both boys and girls.

Turner's syndrome (XO) is not associated with general learning difficulties although performance IQ is slightly below average. It occurs only in girls.

107. E There is a fault in the breakdown of heparin sulphate.

Sanfilippo's syndrome is an autosomal recessive disorder with four enzymatically different forms that are involved with the breakdown pathway of heparin sulphate. All are associated with progressive learning disability. The reported prevalence has varied from 1 in 25 000 to 1 in 324 617.

The clinical features associated with this syndrome include: severe learning disability with mild somatic features, which include moderately severe claw hand, mild dwarfism, hypertrichosis, hearing loss, mild hepatosplenomegaly, biconvex dorsolumbar vertebrae and mild joint stiffness.

The common behavioural problems include: restlessness, destructiveness, aggression and sleep problems.

The prognosis is poor and many die of chest infection by the age of 10–20.

108. A Catatonic features are common.

The symptoms of psychosis in this population tend to be florid but banal. Ideas that have been influenced by radio and the television are found frequently. Impulsive, aggressive and unpredictable behaviours may dominate the clinical picture. Making a diagnosis of schizophrenia in someone who is learning disabled is challenging due to verbal communication difficulties.

Short-term psychotic states are found relatively frequently among learning-disabled adolescents and young adults.

There is an increased prevalence of psychotic disorder in people with learning disability compared with the general population.

109. A Approximately two-thirds of cases of visual impairment go unnoticed by carers.

The prevalence of sensory impairment (visual and hearing) is much greater in adults with intellectual disability than in the general population. Hearing impairment is at least 40% higher whereas visual impairment is at least 8.5% higher. It has been found that >90% of people with severe and profound intellectual disability had visual impairment whereas nearly two-thirds of cases go unnoticed.

Rubella can cause sensorineural congenital hearing loss, central auditory imperceptions, visual impairment and developmental delay.

Usher's syndrome is the most common cause of deaf–blindness in adults, causing 5–10% of cases of congenital hearing loss and >50% of cases of deaf–blindness. An association between Usher's syndrome and psychosis has been reported in up to 23%.

110. E Ordering

The prevalence of obsessive–compulsive disorder in the learning–disabled population is 2.5%. Intellectually disabled clients may find difficulty articulating their obsessional thoughts, and compulsive acts are readily observed. Unlike the general population, in whom hand washing, checking and cleaning are commonly observed, these compulsions are less common in adult learning-disabled population, with ordering being the most common compulsion.

111. B Down's syndrome

This affects up to 1 in 600 births with older mothers at much greater risk. This is the most common single cause of severe generalised learning disability, accounting for up to a third of all cases. Of people with the condition, 95% are due to an extra chromosome 21, resulting from non-disjunction, which is more common in older mothers. There is an increased risk later in life of deafness, leukaemia and Alzheimer's disease

112. B Hunter's syndrome

This is an X-linked recessive condition mapped to Xq27–28. It is caused by iduronate sulphate deficiency. The incidence is 1:132 000 to 1:280 000. It is more common in Ashkenazi Jews (1:34 000).

- Type A: progressive learning difficulties and physical disability with death before age 15
- Type B: milder form with minimal intellectual impairment and better prognosis.

Clinical features: dyostosis (dwarfism, grotesque facies, degenerative hip disease, joint stiffness, claw hand, pes cavus, cervical cord compression), eye defects (retinitis pigmentosa, papilloedema, hypertrichosis) and umbilical/inguinal hernia.

Hurler's syndrome and phenylketonuria are autosomal recessive disorders. Neurofibromatosis is an autosomal dominant disorder.

113. D Most perpetrator programmes are influenced by feminist theory.

Epidemiology related to domestic abuse shows that one in four women experiences abuse at least once in her lifetime, with the annual incidence rate being 10%. Of victims 47% would disclose to a relative or friend. The police would be the next to hear about the incident (20%) followed by medical staff (10%). Since 1992, the Domestic Violence Intervention Project (DVIP) has been running programmes for perpetrators of domestic violence. These are group programmes based on cognitive–behavioural theory. Group programmes reduce denial, help to develop positive social attitudes and develop support systems.

114. B The majority of male first offenders do not reoffend after their conviction.

Indecent exposure or exhibitionism is a non-indictable sexual offence, and therefore most cases are managed in the magistrates' courts in England and Wales. Of first offenders 80% are said not to reoffend and the court appearance alone has a deterrent effect. The personality characteristics of exhibitionists are summarised as: timidity of character; lack of social skills; difficulty in anger control; poor psychosexual adjustment; and a history of minor criminal offences. Most exposers do so at times of personal stress, are more likely to be married and do not show the characteristics of other sexual offenders. The use of anti-libidinal drugs such as cyproterone acetate may be appropriate in those few aggressive exhibitionists whose behaviour is escalating dangerously. Over 80% of exhibitionists show two or more different paraphilias. The perpetrators usually make no attempt to enter into any kind of relationship with the victim.

115. A The children do not have a genuine underlying illness

The mothers have a high incidence of somatoform disorders. Munchausen's syndrome by proxy (also known as factitious illness by proxy) covers the syndrome of a parent deliberately creating an impression that her or his child is ill. The presentation can be in any bodily system, but common forms are factitious epilepsy, non-accidental poisoning and apparent life-threatening events in infancy or multisystem disorders. It may present in children who do have a genuine underlying illness. The perpetrator will frequently have had nursing experience.

- Most perpetrators are female, 79% of whom have a somatisation disorder themselves and half have a personality disorder, particularly so among fabricators who induce illness.
- The mortality rate for children is between 5 and 10%.
- Unusually families are often intact, although 40% have serious marital problems.

116. B Mentally ill mothers

In a study based on a 6-year cohort of 89 women examined in a remand prison, six groups of maternal filicide (the killing by a mother of her own child aged >12 months) were identified (**Table 2.6**).

Table 2.6 Definitions of injuries to children		
Fatal non-accidental injury	40%	These mothers had chaotic personal and social backgrounds with unstable lifestyles and relationships. Some had personality disorder, low intelligence and depressed mood
Mentally ill mothers	27%	Including psychotic illness, major depression and personality disorder with depressed mood sufficient to warrant inpatient care. In some cases there was more than one victim and simultaneous suicidal ideation or actions were usual
Neonaticides	12%	Killing of a baby within 24 hours of birth. Psychiatric disorder was not a factor. They were younger than the other filicides and were usually attempting to conceal an unwanted birth
Retaliating mothers	10%	These were said to be mothers directing misplaced aggression from a partner towards the child victim. They had significant personality disorders and were said to be using the child to manipulate her partner
Killing unwanted children	9%	This group of mothers received diagnoses of antisocial personality disorder or were immature women living apart from partners and beset by social problems
Mercy killing	1 case	This was the killing of a suffering disabled child

117. D Presence of violent sexual fantasies

Risk factors for sexual reoffending are as follows:

- Static factors: forensic history, history of past offences, number and type
- Personality factors: dissocial/psychopathic personality characterised by poor interpersonal skills, poor social support and poor emotion control.

118. D Structured professional judgement has been shown to be a valid approach.

Structured professional judgement tools utilise the best features of actuarial and clinical approaches, and they have been proven to be both useful and valid. Actuarial tools still have a role in aiding decision-making. However, they should not be used alone when determining the risk of violence. Neglecting the influence of contextual factors on the likelihood of particular outcomes has long been noted as a source of error in risk assessment.

119. E The rate is approximately eight to nine times that found in the general population.

The annual rate has doubled in the last 7 years. It is the most common mode of death in prison. It almost always happens by hanging. Suicide is most common in remand prisoners. Suicides do not differ in antecedents from a general prison population. The suicide risk in prison is often managed by isolation of the prisoner.

120. A Diazepam

All the options given are relevant in the context of substance misuse. However, with a substance-induced intoxication state, the important treatment is control, so the immediate treatment consists of administration of the benzodiazepine.

However, talking down a patient for the remainder of the trip is time-consuming and potentially hazardous, given the lability of the patient's condition. The patient is treated with diazepam 20 mg orally which stops panic attacks in about 20 min. Treatment with diazepam should be considered superior to 'talking down'. Haloperidol can be used in severe intoxication for a limited time. Intoxication usually lacks withdrawal symptoms.

121. A Intellectual disability

Fetal alcohol syndrome is a congenital syndrome affecting newborns when there is history of harmful use of alcohol or alcohol dependence in the pregnant mother. Its features include intellectual disability, small stature, low birthweight, limb defects, cleft palate, thin upper lip and smooth philtrum, and hyperactivity.

122. D Methadone: 36 hours

Table 2.7 Approximate half-life of drugs of misuse

Drug	Half-life
Heroin	2 min
Cocaine	1 h
Codeine, morphine	3 h
MDMA	6 h
Temazepam	10 h
Amphetamines	12 h
Cannabis	20 h
Methadone	36 h
Diazepam	48 h

123. D The onset of withdrawal symptoms may begin up to 10 days after birth.

The common symptoms of opioid neonatal abstinence syndrome include gastrointestinal disturbances, irritability, hyperactivity, feeding and sleep disturbances, and autonomic hyperactivity. Withdrawal symptoms usually begin 24–72 hours after birth but can be delayed up to 10 days. Depending on the severity of dependence, 50–90% of neonates will have withdrawal symptoms. Lethargy and reduced muscle tone are seen in the floppy baby syndrome.

124. E Splitting

This is found most frequently in those with borderline personality disorder. It occurs when people, both past and present, are divided into their polar opposites. Thus, they are regarded as perfect or deeply flawed, exclusively nurturing or rejecting.

- Denial is the expressed refusal to acknowledge a threatening reality.
- Displacement is the process by which interest and/or emotion is shifted from one object onto another less threatening one, so that the latter replaces the former.
- Projection is the defence against unpalatable anxieties, impulses or attributes in one's own psyche, which are attributed to an external origin.
- Repression overlaps with denial. It is characterised by the unconscious forgetting of painful ideas or impulses in order to protect the psyche.

125. B Charles Bonnet syndrome

This is characterised by visual hallucinations without any other psychotic features or any evidence of psychiatric disorder. It is associated with visual impairment. The content of the hallucinations varies from straight lines to complex pictures of people and buildings. They may be enjoyable or distressing. Its importance for psychiatrists lies in not making an erroneous diagnosis of a psychiatric disorder.

126. C Ganser's syndrome

This was first described in 1898 when it was observed in four criminals. Ganser's syndrome continues to have an association with prisoners and army personnel under severe stress, such as awaiting trial or going to war. The person seems to mimic his or her own view of what constitutes severe psychiatric illness.

It is characterised by the following:

- Approximate answers (an answer indicating that the question is understood but the answer is incorrect or absurd)
- Clouding of consciousness with disorientation
- Hallucinations (either auditory or visual)
- Amnesia for the period during the episode.

Perseveration, echolalia, echopraxia and hysterical paralysis may also be observed and symptoms are worse when the patient is being observed.

127. C Group psychotherapy

To varying degrees, Yalom's therapeutic factors are likely to be relevant to all models of group psychotherapy. They include instillation of hope, altruism, universality, collective recapitulation of primary family group, imparting information, group cohesiveness, catharsis and existential factors.

128. A Factitious disorder

A chronic factitious disorder with physical symptoms is sometime known as Munchausen's syndrome or hospital addiction syndrome. It is an important part of the condition by which the patient seeks and achieves hospital treatment by deception. It is characterised by wilful induction or feigning of symptoms (physical and/or psychological), assuming a sick role and the absence of external incentives, e.g. money, avoiding legal responsibility or enhancing physical wellbeing.

129. E Voyeurism

Table 2.8 ICD-10 disorders of gender, sexual preference and development		
F64: gender identity disorders	**F65: disorders of sexual preference**	**Psychological and behavioural disorders associated with sexual development and orientation**
Transsexualism Dual role transvestism Gender identity of childhood	Fetishism Fetishistic transvestism Exhibitionism Voyeurism Paedophilia Sadomasochism Multiple disorders of sexual preference	Sexual maturation disorder Ego: dystonic sexual orientation Sexual relationship disorder

130. E Symptoms become more pronounced in the evenings.

Ekbom's syndrome is also known as delusional parasitosis or monosymptomatic hypochondriacal psychosis. Usually the patient presents with isolated delusions concerned with ideas of skin infested with bugs. The incidence increases with age and is equal in both men and women. The prevalence is 1–1.5%.

Answers: EMIs

131. A Confounder
Drug use is a confounder and independently associated with both mental illness and crime.

132. F Specificity
The test correctly identified all the people who did not have agoraphobia.

133. C Intention-to-treat analysis
Imputation gives the last value the average of the previous values. This is to analyse the data for drop-outs and to reduce bias.

134. A Binary data
The statistical data can be divided into continuous (dimensional) or categorical (discrete). Age and height are examples of continuous data. The categorical data are further divided into binary, nominal and ordinal. Dead or alive is an example of binary data, which means that only two mutually exclusive categories are present.

135. F Ratio data
In nominal data, three or more unique categories bear no mathematical relationship to each other but they are coded for the purpose of analysis. The ordinal data would have features of nominal data and, on the top of this, they would have an order inherent in the measurement scale, but they are not quantifiable, e.g. socioeconomic class.

136. C Interval data
This is useful when the difference between the points is equal across the scale, e.g. Fahrenheit scale. In ratio data there are features of interval data, but they also have a true zero, e.g. in the centigrade or Celsius scale.

137. H Piblokto
This is a culture-bound syndrome seen in the Arctic region. It is characterised by an abrupt episode of a dissociative nature and includes features such as tearing off clothing, breaking furniture, shouting obscenities and extreme excitement for about half an hour. It is generally followed by a seizure. Later the person does not remember the episode.

138. E Dhat
This is encountered on the Indian subcontinent and is characterised by feelings of weakness, lethargy and exhaustion. It is attributed to the loss of semen as a result of excessive masturbation because semen is considered to be a precious resource of energy.

139. C Bouffée délirante

This is a culture-specific syndrome commonly seen in African–Caribbean populations. In ICD-10, it is classified under acute and transient psychotic disorders. The presenting symptoms are sudden onset of psychomotor excitement, agitation and aggression. The patient will also be confused. There may be hallucinations or paranoid delusions.

Table 2.9 Culture-bound syndromes

Syndrome	Country/Culture	Clinical features
Koro	South and east Asia	Sudden and intense anxiety of the penis (or vulva) retracting or disappearing
Brain fag	West Africa	Experienced by students in response to the stress of schooling. Difficulty in memory, thinking, concentration, brain fatigue and somatic symptoms
Amok	Malaysia	Amok in Malay means 'mad with uncontrollable rage'. It is a dissociative disorder presenting with sudden outbursts of aggressive and homicidal behaviour. It is believed to be due to an evil spirit entering the body
Ataque de nervios	Latinos from the Caribbean	An idiom of distress – includes uncontrollable shouting, attacks of crying, trembling and heat in the chest rising into the head, aggression, and a sense of being out of control. It often follows a stressful event related to the family

140. C Gerstmann–Sträussler–Scheinker syndrome

This is an extremely rare inherited prion disease caused by autosomal dominant mutations of a prion protein gene. It is a neurodegenerative disorder characterised by ataxia, coordination difficulties, dysarthria and spasticity. As the disease progresses, the patients develop dementia.

141. D Kuru

This had reached epidemic proportions among a defined population living in the Eastern Highlands of Papua New Guinea. It was transmitted by ritual cannibalism. It has virtually disappeared since the practice was abolished in the 1950s.

142. B Creutzfeldt–Jakob disease

Human prion diseases are also known as the subacute spongiform encephalopathies. They are Creutzfeldt–Jakob disease (CJD), Gerstmann–Sträussler syndrome and kuru. The core clinical syndrome of classic CJD is a rapidly progressive multifocal dementia, usually with myoclonus. A small number of cases are inherited as an autosomal dominant disorder due to point or length mutations in the PrP gene. Sporadic CJD affects both sexes equally. New variant CJD was first identified in the UK in 1996. It is linked to bovine spongiform encephalopathy (BSE) and by the same prion strain from contaminated beef products.

143. B Charles Bonnet syndrome

This was first described by Charles Bonnet in 1760. It is usually seen in elderly people, and the prevalence is increased in people with visual impairment. The clinical features include visual loss and visual hallucinations in the absence of cognitive dysfunction. The visual hallucinations of Charles Bonnet syndrome can also occur in the absence of blindness or visual impairment and the usual theme is 'lilliputian hallucinations'. The person has insight and there is no other psychopathology. If visual impairment is due to a treatable condition, treatment of the visual impairment ameliorates the hallucinations.

144. D Diogenes' syndrome

This is also known as senile squalor syndrome, and is commonly seen in elderly people. The clinical features include severe self-neglect, isolation and withdrawal, compulsive hoarding and lack of insight. There is no other primary psychopathology such as depression or psychosis. Patients with frontal lobe damage are at a higher risk of developing this syndrome. These patients live in homes with poor conditions and resist treatment. Prognosis is poor.

145. C Dementia with Lewy bodies

Diffuse Lewy body disease or dementia of Lewy body type is a common form of dementia in the elderly population. The core clinical features include dementia, features of parkinsonism and visual hallucinations. Patients present with antipsychotic hypersensitivity, orthostatic hypertension and frequent falls. Confusion and excessive daytime sleepiness are also seen in these patients.

146. B Delirium unspecified

Delirium not induced by alcohol or other psychoactive substances is a non-specific syndrome. It is characterised by concurrent disturbances of consciousness, attention, concentration, perception, thinking, memory, mood and sleep–wake cycle. It may occur at any age but is more common after the age of 60. It is accompanied by psychomotor and emotional disturbances. Most patients recover within ≤ 4 weeks; however, some patients may take up to 6 months to recover from the delirium.

147. A Alzheimer's dementia

This is the most common form of dementia in presenile groups, i.e. aged <65, and senile groups, i.e. aged >65. Frontotemporal dementia and prion disease are relatively more common whereas vascular dementia is uncommon. A high proportion of cases are due to genetic factors. MMSE has a specificity and sensitivity for dementia of approximately of 80%, when a cut-off score of 23 out of 30 is chosen.

148. C Depressive peudo-dementia

This means that some retarded, depressed patients have conspicuous difficulty in concentration and remembering. However, a careful cognitive testing reveals no major defect of memory. Depressive symptoms usually predate the memory deficits. 'Don't know' responses and poor involvement with cognitive tests are characteristic of depressive pseudo-dementia.

149. K Rivastigmine

Dementia occurs in up to 40% of cases of Parkinson's disease, especially later-onset cases and in patients with severe bradykinesia. L-Dopa does not improve dementia in these patients. Rivastigmine may help patients with mild-to-moderate dementia.

150. J Risperidone

Behavioural and psychological symptoms such as psychosis, agitation and mood swings affect 50–80% patients to varying degrees. Both first- and second-generation antipsychotics are associated with increased mortality and cerebrovascular accidents. Risperidone is the only drug licensed in the UK for managing behavioural and psychological symptoms in dementia. It should be used on a short-term basis (up to 6 weeks) in moderate-to-severe Alzheimer's disease when non-pharmacological approaches have been exhausted.

151. G Memantine

Memantine is licensed in the UK for the treatment of moderately severe to severe Alzheimer's disease. It is a glutamate receptor antagonist at NMDA receptors. This action is considered neuroprotective and disease modifying. Memantine can be used in patients who are unable to take anticholinesterases.

152. A Autistic disorders, D Hyperactivity disorder, H Tic disorders

L Kanner first described autism (autistic disturbances of affect contact) in 1943. He emphasised two essential diagnostic features: autism and difficulties with change. He also noted atypical language in autistic disorders. He had assumed that the autistic children had the potential for normal intelligence. Autism is frequently associated with intellectual disability. The estimated prevalence of autism is 13 per 10 000, Asperger's syndrome is 4 per 10 000 and atypical autism is 1 per 150. The ratio of autism in boys and girls is 3.5–4: 1. This ratio varies with IQ level, i.e. females with autism and IQ in the normal range are probably 20 times less common than males. The reasons for the sex difference are unclear. It is assumed that the degree of insult required to produce autism in females must be greater than for males.

Hyperkinetic disorder describes a constellation of overactivity, impulsivity and inattentiveness. These core problems often coexist with other difficulties of learning, behaviour or mental life. Its prevalence depends on the cut-off point chosen, which depends on the diagnostic criteria and the cultural attitudes of raters. It varies from 2.4% to 9% in children. Boys are two to three times more affected than girls. In adults it is estimated to be 4%.

Tics are sudden, rapid, non-rhythmic, stereotyped, repetitive movements (motor tics) or sounds (vocal tics). The motor tics can be simple (e.g. neck jerking, eye blinking, elevation of shoulders) or complex, in which simple tics involve facial movements, jumping, gyrating, touching, kicking, grooming behaviour or echo kinesis (repeating someone's movement). Simple vocal tics include throat clearing, sniffing, sucking air, grunting, snorting, humming or barking. Complex vocal tics include echolalia, palilalia and coprolalia (socially inappropriate utterances). About 18% of boys and 11% of girls manifest some form of tics.

153. C Depression (pre-pubertal), E School refusal, F Selective mutism

The point prevalence of depression in prepubertal children is about 1–2% and about 3–8% in adolescents. The prevalence of bipolar affective disorder is about 1%. The male:female ratio for prepubertal depression is approximately 1:1.

The term 'school refusal' is no longer used in current approaches. It is included in separation anxiety disorder (SAD). The key feature of SAD is presentation of anxiety related to the fear that harm will befall an attachment figure. SAD represents the most common anxiety disorder in children with a prevalence of about 5% in prepubertal children.

Selective mutism is the persistent refusal to talk in certain situations despite being able to talk in other situations. The most common pattern is talking at home but not at school or other places. The refusal to talk cannot be accounted for by any speech disorder. It is a rare condition with a prevalence of about 0.75–0.80%. It is slightly more common in girls.

154. B Depression (postpubertal), G Specific phobias

The male:female ratio for post-pubertal depression is about 1:3. This may be related to estradiol and testosterone associated with puberty. In contrast, the risk for bipolar affective disorder is equal regardless of puberty.

The key feature of specific phobias is excessive and persistent fear of a specific stimulus or object. They can manifest to a range of objects such as potentially dangerous animals or natural scenarios. It tends to start in early life and is more common in women.

Table 2.10 Prevalence of child and adolescent psychiatric conditions by sex

Marked male excess	Male and females approximately equal	Marked female excess
Autistic disorders Hyperactivity disorders Conduct/oppositional disorders Juvenile delinquency Completed suicide Tic disorders, e.g. Gilles de la Tourette's syndrome Nocturnal enuresis in older children Specific developmental disorders, e.g. language and reading disorders	Depression (pre-pubertal) Selective mutism School refusal	Specific phobias, e.g. insects Diurnal enuresis Deliberate self-harm (postpubertal) Anorexia nervosa Bulimia nervosa

155. B 1–3 months

The following are the approximate times of various personal and social milestones:

- Sleeps and feeds – newborn
- May smile back at parent or examiner – 1–2 months
- Smiles spontaneously – 1.5–3 months
- Finger feeds – 4–8 months
- Smiles at self in mirror – 4–8 months
- Chewing – 5–7 months
- Shy with strangers – 5–10 months
- Drinks from cup – 6–16 months
- Takes off clothes – 14–20 months
- Dry during day – 18–38 months
- Separates easily from mother – 20–50 months
- Uses knife and fork – 32–50 months

156. D 5–10 months

As memory develops in the first year of life, and as the infant becomes more able to express emotion and move independently, so there is evidence for selective attachment. This is shown from around 6–8 months onwards by the upset caused by leaving the attachment figure, by seeking his or her comfort when feeling threatened and by a general wariness of strangers.

157. F 18–36 months

In normal development, the age at which children acquire bladder control is variable. Most children of normal intelligence and health can successfully reach toilet training during the daytime and use it appropriately without wetting themselves by the age of 4. By the fifth birthday only 1% have troublesome daytime wetting. Children generally achieve urinary control by day before the night.

158. G Right temporal lobe focus

Speech automatism, and recurrent, irrelevant and emotionally toned utterances occur due to disturbance of the right temporal lobe focus.

159. D Left temporal lobe focus

Transient dysphasia occurs due to disturbance in the left temporal lobe focus.

160. H Temporal lobe epilepsy (TLE)

Compulsion to think on restricted topics such as religiosity, eternity, death, also called forced thinking, is seen in temporal lobe epilepsy.

161. H Temporal lobe epilepsy

The whole episode from the patient's past life is relived in a brief period of time as a complex organised experience. Panoramic memory is seen in TLE. Sudden fear and intense anxiety without any provocation also occurs in TLE.

162. I Parietal lobe test

The parietal lobe has a number of functions which include left–right orientation. Tests for right–left orientation involve asking the patient to raise his or her left or right hand. Furthermore, this can be done by asking the patient to touch his or her left ear with the right hand. Constructional apraxia can be demonstrated by asking the patient to copy interlocking pentagons.

163. C Attention and concentration

Serial sevens is a part of both the MMSE and Addenbrooke's examination as a test of attention and concentration. The patient is asked to subtract 7 from 100, and this is done a total of 5 times, giving a score out of 5.

164. F Frontal lobe test

The go–no-go test is another frontal lobe test in which the patient is asked to respond to a cue; it tests sustained attention. Examples include asking the patient to lift the finger on hearing a tapping sound and subsequently to drop the finger after hearing two tapping sounds.

165. C Cannabis

Regular heavy use of cannabis can sometimes lead to symptoms of low drive, indifference to rewards, contented lethargy, diffuse thinking and poor concentration. This amotivational syndrome can arise from cannabis toxicity.

166. A Alcohol

Alcohol consumption is associated with morbid jealousy, alcoholic hallucinosis, paranoia, depression, sexual dysfunction, subdural haematomas and the Wernicke–Korsakoff syndrome. Fixed delusions require abstention and a period of treatment with a major tranquilliser in hospital inpatient settings.

167. G Opioids

Neonatal abstinence syndrome is commonly seen in pregnant women who are addicted to opioids. The symptoms include gastrointestinal disturbances, irritability, hyperactivity, feeding and sleep disturbances and autonomic hyperactivity. Withdrawal symptoms usually begin 24–72 hours after birth but can be delayed up to 10 days.

168. E Not guilty by reason of insanity

The finding of not guilty by reason of insanity is a special verdict. In such cases, it is argued that the defendant cannot be held responsible for his actions because of the severity of his mental illness. In this case, it could be argued he did not know that it was wrong to kill in his godly status, and the belief that his neighbour was the devil justified his behaviour. The accused has to prove in a higher court, on the balance of probabilities, that:

- At the time of the offence he laboured under such defect of the mind that he met McNaughton's rules 1843.
- As a result of a defect of reason from disease of the mind he did not know the nature or quality of the act (he did not realise what he was physically doing at the time)
- Due to disease of the mind he did not know what he was doing was wrong
- Where a person is under an insane delusion that prevents the true appreciation of the nature and quality of his act. He therefore has the same degree of responsibility as if the facts were as he imagined them to be.

The above has to be proven on the balance of probabilities and the burden of proof lies with the defence.

169. D Not fit to plead

The principle of being unfit to plead is also known as being under disability. The tests of disability are from the case of a deaf mute (R vs Pritchard 1836). The defendant must have the capacity to:

- Understand the charge
- Instruct a lawyer
- Challenge a juror
- Plead to the charge (guilty or not guilty)
- Understand the evidence.

170. C Insane automatism

This patient clearly has a history of epilepsy and it could be argued that his behaviour resulted in his body not being under the control of his mind.

An automatism is an act committed during a state of unconsciousness or grossly impaired consciousness. It is an unconscious involuntary action and is a defence because the mind does not go with what is being done.

Insane automatism is due to internal causes of behaviour without voluntary control. It is viewed as an event due to a disease of the mind, which is likely to recur, and requires control of that individual to ensure public safety. Examples include epilepsy, insulinoma (causing episodes of hypoglycaemia), and sleepwalking and degenerative brain disease. A successful plea of insane automatism would lead the subject being found not guilty by reason of insanity and therefore McNaughton's rules apply.

171. A Diminished responsibility

The term 'diminished responsibility' was introduced in Section 2 of the Homicide Act 1957. It applies only to murder. Diminished responsibility in essence refers to sentencing where the crime of 'murder' is reduced to 'manslaughter'. It applies to offenders with abnormal state of mind where at the time of killing the offender suffers from a state of mind that is different from a reasonable man with a normal mind. It is a legal concept rather than a medical one.

Not all defendants experiencing psychosis automatically satisfy the criteria. The diminished responsibility criteria have recently been revised in England and Wales. They were first introduced in the 1957 Homicide Act. Section 52 of the Coroners and Justice Act 2009 replaces this and applies to all defendants charged with murder taking place on or after 4 October 2010.

172. D Kruskal–Wallis test

For variables that are not normally distributed non-parametric tests are used: Wilcoxon's rank sum test is used for paired data, the Mann–Whitney U-test for two independent groups and the Kruskal–Wallis test for three or more groups.

173. C Friedman's test

This is used in comparing three or more paired samples when data are skewed/discrete numerical/ranked categorical. χ^2 test is used to compare the proportions of discrete variables belonging to two or more samples. If the sample size is very small the χ^2 test cannot be applied. In these situations, Fisher's exact test is used.

174. A ANOVA test

This is used when three or more groups are normally distributed.

175. B χ^2 test

This is a non-parametric test for non-normally distributed data. It compares expected frequencies with observed frequencies of categorical data.

176. H Wilcoxon's signed rank test

This is a non-parametric test for non-normally distributed data. It is used for measuring the difference between two-paired samples.

177. F Matched pairs Student's *t*-test

Student's *t*-test is a parametric test that compares the means in two normally distributed groups. There are two types: an independent *t*-test in which the two groups are different participants and the paired *t*-test which the two groups have the same participants at different time points.

Answers: EMIs

178. D Post-concussion syndrome

This is also called post-traumatic syndrome. It is characterised by a constellation of symptoms that may result in surprisingly severe disability after mild head injury.

179. B Dysprosody

This is a phenomenon where the normal rhythms and intonations of speech are lost, more so after right hemisphere damage. This interferes with social communication because the voice sounds flat and fails to convey emotion.

180. E Reduplicative paramnesia

This is the most pathognomonic of brain injury and is also associated with postictal confusional states. The term 'reduplicative paramnesia' covers a range of phenomena, which are often observed concurrently. An example of the phenomenon could be any delusion involving duplication, e.g. that events have been duplicated or that the patient has a second left leg.

181. F Sensitivity

This is the proportion of people who truly have the disorder (true positives). Sensitivity of a test is a positive test in the proportion of people with the disorder.

182. G Specificity

This is the proportion of people who truly do not have the disorder (true negatives). Specificity of a test is the negative test in the proportion of people without the disorder.

183. D Positive predictive value (PPV)

This is the proportion of people with a positive test who have the disorder. PPV is not a constant property of a test because it rises with an increase in the prevalence of a disorder.

184. C Negative predictive value (NPV)

This is the proportion of people with a negative test who are truly free from the disorder. NPV is not a constant property of a test because it rises with a decrease in the prevalence of the disorder.

185. A Accuracy

This means the exactness or precision of a test. In other words, it is the proportion of correct results including all true positives and true negatives.

186. I Trazodone

This has both antidepressant and sedative properties. It is therefore sometimes used as a hypnotic in elderly people. It acts mainly via the $5HT_{2A}$-receptor and is also used as an anxiolytic. The side effects include falls and oversedation.

187. G Rivastigmine

This is the only cholinesterase inhibitor currently available as a patch preparation. It is produced in doses of 4.6 mg/24 h and 9.5 mg/24 h. The patch may be useful for patients who experience side effects from oral ingestion of cholinesterase inhibitors.

188. F Risperidone

If the persistent aggression in Alzheimer's dementia does not respond to non-pharmacological measures and there is substantial risk of harm to self or others, one should consider using risperidone. It is the only licensed antipsychotic medication in the UK for treating behavioural disturbances and aggression in patients with dementia. It should be given in therapeutic doses for up to 6 weeks.

189. G Rivastigmine

This may be the safest cholinesterase inhibitor to prescribe for patients with pre-existing cardiac disease due to its lack of interaction with other cardiac drugs. One study showed adverse cardiac effects for patients with mild cognitive impairment who were prescribed galantamine.

190. A Donepezil

This is the only short-acting preparation of a cholinesterase inhibitor available as a once-daily dose. Both rivastigmine and galantamine are given twice daily. Galantamine is also available as a long-acting preparation that can be given once daily. In addition, there is a galantamine liquid preparation.

191. G MDMA

This is a synthetic amphetamine that is misused by some people. Any drug in this class has a huge potential for misuse. Acute intoxication with MDMA can present with symptomatology suggestive of serotoninergic syndrome and neuroleptic malignant syndrome (NMS). It is managed along the same lines as NMS. Unfortunately, there is no evidence base for pharmacological treatment of withdrawal symptoms.

192. D γ-Hydroxybutyrate (GHB)

This is an inhalant and its acute intoxication can lead to cardiac arrhythmia or vasovagal inhibition, resulting in cardiac arrest. Its long-term use can lead to multiple organ damage.

193. A Alcohol

This is a natural product of the breakdown of carbohydrates in plants. It has been known to humankind from prehistoric times, and has been used by almost all cultures across the world:

- Cannabis: cannabinoid receptors
- LSD: partial agonist at post-synaptic receptors
- Heroin: acts on opioid receptors, dopaminergic and noradrenergic systems
- Nicotine: agonist at nicotinic subtype of acetylcholine receptors
- Diazepam: GABA-A receptors.

194. A Ceiling effect

This is one of the common sources of misinterpretation of publications. It is a term used when the values of many subjects are on a variable near the maximum possible value, i.e. 'ceiling'. It refers to two distinct meanings: (1) a level at which an independent variable no longer has an effect on a dependent variable, or (2) the level above which variance in an independent variable is no longer measurable. It can be caused by a variety of factors, and it causes a problem for certain types of analysis because it reduces the possible variation in the sample. The floor effect is the opposite of the ceiling effect. This refers to a situation when data cannot take a lower value than a particular number. It is a statistical phenomenon in which most measures fall in a very low range of possible values. It may lead to type 2 error.

195. G Order effect

This is a systematic different between the first and subsequent assessments. It occurs when a test is consistently given before another test, such that any differences between tests may reflect the order in which the tests were administered, rather than any other factors, e.g. time of day or months, etc. Order effects that are associated with passage of time include practice and fatigue effects.

196. H Regression to mean sequential effect

This is the tendency for extreme values of a test to decrease with repeated measurements over time. In other words, if any test is repeated the outliers are likely to tend towards the mean owing to measurement error. It helps to avoid making wrong inferences. It is an important consideration in the design of research experiments. The conditions under which regression to the mean occurs depend on its mathematical definition. It had been historically called reversion to the mean and regression to mediocrity.

197. D Observer bias

This arises when the researchers are not blinded to the participants' status or group membership and unconsciously, or not, tend to alter their approach. It occurs when the observer, i.e. researcher, is influenced by prior knowledge or experience of the situation or participants under investigation. It can be 'exposure suspicion bias', i.e. exposure is measured after the disease, or 'diagnostic suspicion bias' if researchers strive harder to detect disease in those known to have been exposed, or tend to rate outcomes more favourably in the experimental group in an RCT. All observers tend to make observations that concur with their expectations, i.e. 'expectation bias'.

198. G Selection bias

This occurs when there is an error in selecting the participants or groups to participate in a research study. It is also known as selection error. It arises through the identification and/or recruitment of an unrepresentative study population. It is particularly important for descriptive research in observational studies, and potentially important in all research. It can be introduced by the researchers (sampling bias) or the participants (response bias). There are several types of selection bias, e.g. time interval, exposure, studies to be included in meta-analysis, data, attrition and observer selection.

199. C Information bias

This is also called observation or measurement bias and it arises through the systematic and differential misclassification of disease or exposure by both researchers and participants. In addition it is known as cognitive bias because it may involve distorted evaluation of information. Random or non-differential misclassification is not a bias because it is non-systematic, will add only 'noise' and will reduce the strength of the associations.

200. G Selection bias

This arises through the identification and/or recruitment of an unrepresentative study population. It is particularly important for descriptive research in observational studies, and potentially important for any research. It can be introduced by the researchers (sampling bias) or the participants (response bias).

Chapter 3

Mock Exam: 3

Questions: MCQs

For each question, select one answer option

1. A new meaning cannot be understood as arriving from the patient's affective state or previous attitudes. Which of the following refers to the attribution of a new meaning, usually in the sense of self-reference to a normally perceived object?

    A   Delusional misinterpretation
    B   Delusional memory
    C   Delusional mood
    D   Delusional perception
    E   Delusional work

2. Which of the following is correct practice for ECT, according to the Electroconvulsive Therapy Accreditation Service (ECTAS)?

    A   Oxygen is administered before ECT
    B   Patients can go to the ward directly after ECT
    C   The referring psychiatrist can prescribe four or more sessions at a time
    D   There can be up to three ECT sessions routinely provided to patients
    E   Seizure induced can be complex partial or generalised tonic clonic

3. Which of the following is the most appropriate indication for a cohort study?

    A   Multiple exposures
    B   Rare exposures
    C   Single outcome
    D   Studying complex issues
    E   Suitable for a rare disease

4. A 19-year-old man heard babies crying whenever he saw traffic lights changing and was thus convinced that the babies were being harmed by them. Which of the following best describes this phenomenon?

    A   Autoscopy
    B   Extracampine hallucination
    C   Functional hallucination
    D   Reflex hallucination
    E   Secondary hallucination

5. A research method involves plotting the first few digits of numerical observations along a vertical axis and then adding numbers to a single group or two groups to represent individual values of observation. What is the name of this research method?

A   Box-and-whisker plot
B   Dot plot
C   Histogram
D   Scatter plots
E   Stem-and-leaf plot

6. Who wrote the book *Myth of Mental Illness*?

   A   Erving Goffman
   B   Michel Foucault
   C   RD Laing
   D   Sigmund Freud
   E   Thomas Szaz

7. Which of the following economic analyses would you use to compare two preventive treatments for dementia?

   A   Cost–benefit analysis
   B   Cost-effectiveness analysis
   C   Cost-minimisation analysis
   D   Cost–utility analysis
   E   Fiscal impact analysis

8. Which of the following statements about the pharmacological treatment of sex offenders is correct?

   A   Cyproterone acetate causes side effects similar to those of surgical castration.
   B   Cyproterone acetate is a gonadotrophin-releasing hormone agonist.
   C   The side effects of medroxyprogesterone acetate are irreversible.
   D   The selective serotonin reuptake inhibitors (SSRIs) are not as well tolerated as hormonal treatments.
   E   It should be used in place of psychotherapy in high-risk offenders.

9. Which of the following statements about the availability of ECT policies and protocol is correct, according to the Electroconvulsive Therapy Accreditation Service (ECTAS)?

   A   There is no requirement for a maintenance treatment protocol as it is not encouraged
   B   There is no separate requirement for a protocol for treatment of young people under 18 years
   C   Policies relating to ECT must be checked once every 3 years
   D   Protocol for neuroleptic malignant syndrome should be available
   E   Protocol for storing Dantrolene should be available

10. In a study, sensitivity is 92% and specificity 94%. What is the likelihood ratio of a positive test result?

    A   0.47
    B   1.06
    C   1.86
    D   11.75
    E   15.33

11. A 81-year-old man was admitted after a stroke. The neurologist suspected that he was depressed. Which of the following symptoms suggests depression in the presence of a stroke?

    A   Anorexia
    B   Feeling punished
    C   Lethargy

D Psychomotor retardation
E Weight loss

12. A 56-year-old man was admitted after a myocardial infarction. He was diagnosed with depression. Which of the following antidepressants is likely to be the first choice?

   A Agomelatine
   B Dothiepin
   C Lithium
   D Sertraline
   E Venlafaxine

Use the following information to answer questions 13–16

A new screening test was used to diagnose schizophrenia in 90 psychotic patients. The data in **Table 3.1** were observed.

Screening test	Gold standard	
	Schizophrenia positive	Schizophrenia negative
Positive test	80 (a)	10 (b)
Negative test	20 (c)	70 (d)

Table 3.1 Screening test for schizophrenia

13. What is the positive predictive value?

   A 0.11
   B 0.22
   C 0.28
   D 0.77
   E 0.88

14. What is the negative predictive value?

   A 0.55
   B 0.66
   C 0.77
   D 0.88
   E 0.99

15. What is the likelihood ratio for a positive test (LR+)?

   A 4.15
   B 5.15
   C 6.15
   D 7.15
   E 8.15

16. What is the likelihood ratio for a negative test (LR–)?

   A 0.11
   B 0.22
   C 0.77
   D 0.88
   E 6.15

Mock Exam: 3

For each question, select one answer option

17. A 32-year-old man with HIV infection was worried about the brain complications of his condition. What is the most common CNS complication of HIV disease (AIDS)?

    A   Cerebral vasculitis
    B   HIV encephalitis
    C   HIV leukoencephalopathy
    D   HIV-associated dementia
    E   Primary non-Hodgkin's malignant lymphoma of CNS

18. In which of the following personality disorders is the self-serving attributional bias exaggerated?

    A   Anankastic personality disorder
    B   Anxious (avoidant) personality disorder
    C   Emotionally unstable personality disorder
    D   Paranoid personality disorder
    E   Schizoid personality disorder

19. What was the outcome of the CUtLASS study and its subsequent economic analysis?

    A   Atypical antipsychotics were less than 50% likely to be cost-effective.
    B   Atypical antipsychotics were associated with quality of life.
    C   Conventional antipsychotics had a higher cost.
    D   Conventional antipsychotics had lower quality-adjusted life years (QALYs).
    E   The primary outcome measure was quality of life.

20. A 40-year-old man started to follow and attempted to contact his ex-girlfriend repeatedly in such an intrusive manner that she felt scared and was frightened to go out on her own. Which of the following statements about the victims of stalking by someone who was previously known is correct?

    A   Victims are usually stalked for shorter periods of time.
    B   Victims are at a less risk of physical violence.
    C   Victims are unlikely to suffer from major distress.
    D   Victims are less likely to feel guilt.
    E   Victims are often not believed by others.

21. What is the probable risk of agranulocytosis with clozapine treatment in the UK?

    A   <1:1000
    B   <1:2000
    C   <1:3000
    D   <1:4000
    E   <1:5000

22. Which of the following relates to falsification of memory occurring in clear consciousness in association with organic pathology?

    A   Confabulation
    B   False memory
    C   Pseudologica fantastica
    D   Retrospective falsification
    E   *Vorbeireden*

23. What is the approximate risk of fatal pulmonary embolism with clozapine treatment?

    A   1:2000
    B   1:2500

C   1:3000
D   1:4000
E   1:4500

Use Table 3.2 to answer questions 25–32

Table 3.2 A 2 × 2 table for questions 25–32

Depression identified by two-item screening questionnaire	ICD-10 diagnosis of depression Yes	ICD-10 diagnosis of depression No	Total
Yes	45	50	95
No	5	85	90
Total	50	135	185

25. What is the sensitivity of a two-item screening questionnaire using both items?
    A   60%
    B   70%
    C   80%
    D   90%
    E   100%

26. What is the specificity of the two-item screening questionnaire?
    A   53%
    B   63%
    C   75%
    D   85%
    E   95%

27. What is the predictive power of a positive test using a two-item screening questionnaire?
    A   37%
    B   47%
    C   57%
    D   67%
    E   77%

28. What is the predictive power of a negative test using a two-item screening questionnaire?
    A   55%
    B   64%
    C   74%
    D   85%
    E   94%

29. What is the likelihood ratio of a negative test (LR−) for the two-item screening questionnaire?
    A   0.6
    B   0.16
    C   0.26
    D   0.36
    E   0.46

30. What is the pre-test probability of a two-item screening questionnaire?

    A   7%
    B   17%
    C   27%
    D   37%
    E   47%

31. What is the false-positive rate for the two-item screening questionnaire?

    A   17%
    B   27%
    C   37%
    D   47%
    E   57%

32. What is the false-negative rate for a two-item screening questionnaire?

    A   5%
    B   10%
    C   15%
    D   20%
    E   25%

For each question, select one answer option.

33. A 31-year-old man was recently diagnosed with human immunodeficiency virus (HIV) infection. He would like to learn more about his condition. Which of the following statements about the HIV is correct?

    A   The AIDS–dementia complex or HIV-associated dementia is secondary to opportunistic infections of the central nervous system.
    B   Bacterial infections are common.
    C   The most common CNS neoplasm is secondary non-Hodgkin's malignant lymphoma, occurring in around 2–6% of patients.
    D   The nervous system is a late target in HIV infection.
    E   Progressive encephalopathy in children is due to primary HIV infection of the CNS.

34. Which of the following statements about pathological laughing and crying (PLC) is correct?

    A   PLC is not associated with more depressive, anxious and aggressive behaviours compared with people do not have PLC.
    B   PLC is an essential part of the pseudo-bulbar palsy syndrome.
    C   PLC is usually triggered by a stimulus that would normally trigger the response of laughter or crying.
    D   The prevalence of PLC is approximately 40–50% among patients who have had a stroke.
    E   Tricyclic antidepressants are the first-line treatment.

35. A study was conducted in the general population using a two-item screening questionnaire for depression. A sample of 1500 participants was randomly chosen. It was estimated that the prevalence of depression (ICD-10 categories) was 15%. What is the PPV of this two-item screening questionnaire in the general population?

    A   5%
    B   10%
    C   15%
    D   20%
    E   25%

Questions: MCQs

36. You have met a pharmaceutical representative to discuss a new, recently licensed drug for treatment-resistant schizophrenia. The data showed that the drug prevented annual hospitalisation in 30% more patients than placebo in the RCTs. You wanted to know how many patients you needed to treat (NNT) to prevent hospitalisation. Which of the following is the correct answer?

    A   3
    B   4
    C   5
    D   6
    E   7

37. Which of the following statements about magic mushrooms is correct?

    A   About two to three magic mushrooms are typically used at a time to achieve the effects.
    B   Their abuse is strongly associated with personality disorders.
    C   Management of complications is by benzodiazepines.
    D   They are addictive.
    E   Urine testing can detect the psilocybin constituent of mushrooms.

38. Which one of the following is an adverse effect of phototherapy?

    A   Burning sensation in eyes
    B   Double vision
    C   Headaches
    D   Skin irritation
    E   Skin rashes

39. A 19-year-old man with mild learning disability attended your clinic for a review. His care coordinator who attended with him enquired about the association between epilepsy and learning disability. Which of the following statements about learning disability and epilepsy is correct?

    A   Epilepsy can cause a decline in intellectual functioning.
    B   Learning disability occurs in <10% of people with epilepsy.
    C   Specific causes of epilepsy and learning disability can be identified in most cases.
    D   The presence of epilepsy in the learning-disabled population is approximately 10%.
    E   The prevalence of epilepsy is lower in the more severely disabled than the mildly disabled individuals.

40. A new rating evaluated for major depression had a sensitivity of 90% and a specificity of 90% against the DSM-IV diagnosis. What is the likelihood ratio of a positive result?

    A   3
    B   5
    C   7
    D   9
    E   11

41. The prevalence of anxiety in patients diagnosed with mild cognitive impairment was 20%. An anxiety rating scale with an LR+ of 20 was administered to a patient with mild cognitive impairment. What is the probability that this patient was anxious?

    A   53%
    B   63%
    C   73%
    D   83%
    E   93%

42. A new antidepressant drug was recently licensed. The published data indicated that, in the RCTs, there were two study groups: one using active drug and one using a placebo. Each group consisted of 200 patients. Over a 6-week study period, a 50% drop in the Montgomery–Asberg Depression Rating Scale (MADRS) scores was observed in 80 patients receiving the active drug. However, a similar drop was observed in only 40 patients in the placebo group. What is the NNT from this study for the new antidepressant drug?

    A   3
    B   4
    C   5
    D   6
    E   7

43. Which one of the following conditions is an absolute contraindication for psychosurgery?

    A   Agoraphobia
    B   Alzheimer's disease
    C   Bipolar affective disorder
    D   Persistent delusional disorder
    E   Schizophrenia

44. Which of the following statements about morbid jealousy is correct?

    A   It is associated with high self-esteem.
    B   It is found in ICD-10 as a diagnostic classification.
    C   It is otherwise known as De Clerambault's syndrome.
    D   It may take different psychopathological forms.
    E   It requires that proof of the spouse being faithful is a valid symptom.

45. What should researchers do if there is no information available about the distribution of the data?

    A   Assume normality and use parametric tests
    B   Assume non-normality and use non-parametric tests
    C   Try to modify the data to normal distribution
    D   It doesn't matter because they can use the appropriate test to suit their hypothesis
    E   Expect to provide information as to why no information was available

46. In a sample of 100 people, a test identifies that 91 of them have an illness. Which of the following statements is correct?

    A   The test has a high sensitivity.
    B   The test has a high specificity.
    C   The test has a high positive predictive value.
    D   The test has a high negative predictive value.
    E   The test has high validity.

47. Which of the following statements about the odds ratio is correct?

    A   The odds ratio is also called the cross-product ratio.
    B   An odds ratio of 1 means that there is a 100% of chance of developing a condition.
    C   It is reported in cohort studies.
    D   It is used to calculate the likelihood of developing a condition.
    E   In rare conditions, the odds ratio is more than the risk ratio.

48. A 59-year-man with a 20-year history of bipolar affective disorder attended your outpatient clinic for a review. He would like to discuss the prognosis of his condition. He had heard about rapid cycling mood disorder. Which of the following statements about this disorder is correct?

    A   It has an inherited pattern.
    B   It is usually seen in bipolar II disorder.

C   It is more frequent in males.
D   It is the occurrence of at least three episodes in a year.
E   It occurs in both depression and bipolar disorders.

49. A 14-year-old girl was admitted to the inpatient unit with depressive stupor. She was treated with medication and psychosocial interventions. In the discharge planning meeting, her care coordinator discussed her rights with her. She wanted to discuss 'advanced decision'. Which of the following statements about the legal term 'advanced decision' is true?

   A   A patient can choose to receive a particular treatment under advanced decision
   B   Advance decisions cannot be changed once made
   C   Advance decisions come into force once they are made by the patient
   D   Appropriate treatment may be administered by the responsible clinician even if an advance decision has been made refusing treatment
   E   She can make an advance decision if she has the capacity to understand her illness as well as the treatment process

50. When is the Mantel–Haenszel procedure used?

   A   To calculate the power of the study
   B   To calculate the statistical significance of the study
   C   To combine the studies in a meta-analysis and produce a net effect
   D   To correct for multiple testing
   E   To test for normality of the data

51. In a research study, only the participants did not know which treatment they were receiving. What is this known as?

   A   Cross-over
   B   Double blind
   C   Factorial design
   D   Placebo control
   E   Single blind

52. Which of the following statements about the STEP-BD trial is correct?

   A   All the patients included were not on any baseline mood stabilisers.
   B   Antidepressants have been shown to be efficacious in the management of acute bipolar depression.
   C   Antidepressants were better than placebo at achieving the therapeutic response.
   D   A switch to mania was equal for antidepressants and placebo.
   E   The two antidepressants used in the STEP-BD trial were citalopram and fluoxetine.

53. Which of the following statements about costs is correct?

   A   An opportunity cost is defined as the cost of a decision in terms of the next best alternative; it occurs because human beings have endless needs and require resources to satisfy these needs.
   B   Costs describe the total expenditure in the pursuance of starting the treatment programme.
   C   In the health-provision context, the direct cost of the treatment programme would include all identifiable equipment costs, along with other costs such as project planning, building and premises, staff salaries, equipment administration and so on.
   D   Intangible costs in the health-provision context would include patient-borne costs such as absence from work and other duties during the treatment period, loss of earnings and losses due to treatment side effects.
   E   Intangible costs in the health-provision context would be the value of other things, which are resources used by a treatment programme, that would have been spent in other ways such as other treatment programmes.

54. Which of the following statements about concepts and disorders related to physical complaints is correct?
    A   Accident neurosis is synonymous with post-traumatic neurosis.
    B   Factitious disorder is characterised by physical or psychological symptoms that are feigned for gain.
    C   Patients with hospital addiction syndrome tend to become aggressive and may use sexual elements.
    D   Psychological symptoms are produced intentionally in others in patients with Munchausen's syndrome by proxy.
    E   A sick role is synonymous with Munchausen's syndrome.

55. Which of the following statements about 'risk' as an epidemiological measure is correct?
    A   It is the incidence density.
    B   It is measured in units of case/person time.
    C   It is the percentage of population with time.
    D   It is the cumulative incidence.
    E   It is the rapidity of disease occurrence.

56. Which of the following statements about randomised controlled trials (RCTs) is correct?
    A   They are a study design of choice for prognosis of a disease.
    B   They are conducted when a previous meta-analysis already has a definite result.
    C   They are conducted when a prohibitively high study sample is needed to prove a statistical difference.
    D   They are designed to look at the validation of a screening or diagnostic test.
    E   They include prospective designs.

57. Which of the following is used to determine whether, and to what extent, age, alcohol, smoking and fat intake affect a person's blood sugar levels?
    A   Multiple analysis of variance
    B   Multiple regression using the least-square method
    C   Product–moment correlation coefficient
    D   Regression using the least-square method
    E   Spearman's rank correlation coefficient

58. Which of the following is an appropriate test to compare the heights of boys and girls?
    A   McNemar's test
    B   One-sample (paired) Student's t-test (Wilcoxon's matched-pairs test)
    C   Two-sample (unpaired) Student's t-test (Mann–Whitney U-test)
    D   Two-way analysis of variance (by ranks)
    E χ^2 test

59. Which of the following should be used to determine whether the blood glucose level increases at 30, 60, 90 and 120 min after taking a meal, and whether the increase is different in males and females?
    A   Analysis of variance
    B   Mann–Whitney U-test
    C   Multiple regression analysis
    D   Spearman's rank correlational coefficient
    E   Two-way analysis of variance (by ranks)

60. What is Kaplan–Meier survival analysis?
    A   Comparing various survival indices between two paired groups
    B   Comparing various survival indices among three matched groups

C   Comparing various survival indices among three unmatched groups
D   Comparing various survival indices between two unpaired (independent) groups
E   Looking at various survival indices in one group over the study period

61. Which of the following is used to calculate QALYs?

    A   Cost–benefit analysis
    B   Cost-effective analysis
    C   Cost-minimisation analysis
    D   Cost–utility analysis
    E   Multi-way sensitivity analysis

62. Which of the following introduces the highest probability of bias?

    A   Drop-out events
    B   Last observation carried forward
    C   Missing data analysis
    D   Per-protocol analysis
    E   Sensitivity analysis (the worst-case or best-case scenario)

63. Which of the following measures an internal consistency of a test?

    A   Cronbach's α
    B   Intraclass correlation coefficient
    C   Intrarater reliability
    D κ (Cohen's) statistics
    E   Split-half reliability

64. Which of the following 'endpoints' overcomes the problem of insufficient power in studies?

    A   Clinical endpoint
    B   Composite endpoint
    C   Humane endpoint
    D   Lacunar endpoint
    E   Surrogate endpoint

65. Which of the following can help to reduce type 1 error (i.e. a false-positive result) in a study?

    A   Adjusting the level of the β value in that study
    B   Eliminating confounders
    C   Reducing the heterogeneity in a study sample
    D   Reducing the sample size
    E   Reducing the variance

66. The statistical tests of heterogeneity used in a meta-analysis have a limited statistical power. What are these tests prone to?

    A   They reduce the confidence interval and thus the strength of the study
    B   They show false-positive conclusions with regard to heterogeneity in a meta-analysis
    C   Type 1 error
    D   Type 2 error
    E   Type α error

67. What is a test used to check group differences in the means of two independent groups?

    A χ^2 test
    B   Mann–Whitney test
    C   McNemar's test
    D   Two-sample Student's t-test
    E   Wilcoxon's rank test

Mock Exam: 3

68. A 32-year-old man diagnosed with HIV infection was concerned about complications of his condition. Which of the following statements about opportunistic infections in HIV is correct?

    A   Bacterial invasions are most common.
    B   The most common fungal infection is coccidioidomycosis.
    C   Cytomegalovirus infection causes haemorrhagic encephalitis.
    D   They occur in about 50% of the patients with HIV.
    E   Toxoplasmosis usually presents with focal neurological signs.

69. What is the name of a study in which neither the investigators nor the participants knew what treatment the latter were taking?

    A   Cross-over study
    B   Double-blind study
    C   Factorial design study
    D   Placebo-control study
    E   Single-blind study

70. According to current evidence, how many patients live independently after first-episode schizophrenia?

    A   10%
    B   15%
    C   20%
    D   25%
    E   30%

71. According to ICD-10, what minimum duration of non-organic insomnia meets the diagnostic criteria?

    A   2 weeks
    B   1 month
    C   3 months
    D   6 months
    E   12 months

72. What is the ability to detect true differences between groups known as?

    A α
    B β
    C   Effect size
    D   Power
    E   Probability

73. Combined depression and personality disorders are likely to be associated with poor outcome for depression. What is the likely association according to current evidence?

    A   1-fold
    B   1.5-fold
    C   2-fold
    D   2.5-fold
    E   3-fold

74. A 37-year-old woman was recently diagnosed with obsessive–compulsive disorder (OCD). She is planning to have a family and wanted to know about the risk of OCD in her offspring. Which of the following is a risk factor for developing OCD?

    A   Being a girl
    B   Being married
    C   Depression

D Monozygotic twins with OCD in the other sibling
E Obsessive–compulsive personality disorder

75. A 43-year-old woman with OCD attended your outpatient clinic for a review. She would like to discuss treatment options and her prognosis because she has not been making any progress. Which of the following is associated with a poor prognosis in OCD?

   A Anankastic personality disorder
   B Emotionally unstable personality disorder
   C Paranoid personality disorder
   D Schizoid personality disorder
   E Schizotypal personality disorder

76. An 18-month-old child presented with the following features: facial features (epicanthic folds, microcephaly, short palpebral fissures, underdeveloped philtrum and thin upper lip), growth deficit, central nervous system impairment including hyperactivity and sleep disturbance, optic nerve hypoplasia with poor visual acuity, hearing loss, receptive and expressive language deficits, and cardiac and renal abnormalities. What is the most likely diagnosis?

   A Congenital hypothyroidism
   B Fetal alcohol syndrome
   C Phenylketonuria
   D Rubenstein–Tayebi syndrome
   E Velocardiofacial syndrome

77. A 35-year-old woman was evaluated for excessive daytime sleepiness. Which of the following is least likely to be present?

   A Catalepsy
   B Hypnogogic hallucinations
   C Narcolepsy
   D Sleep apnoea syndrome
   E Sleep paralysis

78. A 48-year-old man presented with a 2-year history of depressed mood, paranoia and recent onset of memory problems. During the assessment, he was fidgeting excessively without any purpose. He did not have any past history of mental health problems. His father had had behavioural problems and unfortunately died in his 40s. What is the most likely diagnosis?

   A Alzheimer's disease of early onset
   B Frontotemporal dementia
   C Gilles de la Tourette's syndrome
   D Huntington's disease
   E Late-onset schizophrenia

79. What is Pfropfschizophrenia?

   A It is another name for undifferentiated schizophrenia.
   B It is schizophrenia in children.
   C It is schizophrenia with learning disability.
   D It is schizophrenia with onset after age 65 years.
   E It is schizophrenia with predominantly negative symptoms.

80. A 37-year-old woman with multiple sclerosis (MS) attended to discuss her prognosis and possible psychiatric aspects of her condition. Which of the following statements about neuropsychiatric presentation in MS is correct?

   A Hysterical reactions are especially common in MS.
   B Intellectual deterioration is rare.
   C Onset of dementia is insidious.

D Psychotic presentations are primarily of a hallucinatory rather than a delusional type.
E Verbal skills are often affected early in the disease process.

81. A 45-year-old man has hyperparathyroidism. He would like to learn more about his condition. Which of the following statements about hyperparathyroidism is correct?

   A The most common cause of hyperparathyroidism is diffuse enlargement of the parathyroid glands.
   B The most common psychiatric presentation is depression with anergia.
   C Diagnosis of hyperparathyroidism is usually made during the early stages of its course.
   D Psychosis occurs in around 25% of patients.
   E The level of calcium does not seem to be related to the severity of the psychiatric symptoms.

82. Which of the following is a Bradford–Hill criterion for causality?

   A Inconsistency
   B Irreversibility
   C Proximity
   D Sensitivity
   E Temporal relationship

83. Which of the following statements about smoking is correct?

   A Children take up smoking for biological reasons.
   B The effect of nicotine on dopamine release is similar to the effect of cocaine.
   C High rates of smoking are seen in couples who do not have children.
   D In the UK, up to 15% of teenagers smoke by the age of 15.
   E Smoking in in women results in halving the risk of ectopic pregnancy.

84. What is the meaning of the term 'pathological alcohol intoxication'?

   A A condition with hallucinations in clear consciousness without autonomic features
   B Consciousness and gait are affected most severely after regular drinking
   C Compulsive drinking
   D Outburst of aggression and uncontrollable rage
   E Refers to a transient state of amnesia due to drinking excessively

85. Which of the following statements about gender is least likely to be correct?

   A A man's positive identity is contingent upon his relationships, care for others and altruistic behaviour.
   B Sex role stereotype makes lifestyle transitions such as marriage and parenthood of different importance for women.
   C The prevalence of mental disorder in men is a third that in women.
   D Women are more likely to experience physical violence and sexual abuse in both childhood and adulthood.
   E Women are more likely to seek psychiatric help and take psychotropic medication.

86. Which of the following statements about late luteal-phase dysphoric disorder is correct?

   A Of women 10% consider them severe enough to seek medical help.
   B During the postmenstrual period, there is an increase in parasuicidal acts.
   C Symptoms are most severe during ovulation.
   D Symptoms improve with age and parity.
   E There is at least a 7-day symptom-free phase after menstruation.

87. In which part of the eye do Kayser–Fleischer rings due to copper deposition occur?

   A Choroid of the eye
   B Cornea of the eye

C   Lens of the eye
D   Retina of the eye
E   Sclera of the eye

88. Which is most likely to be the anatomical location of brain tumours presenting with maximum frequency of neuropsychiatric symptoms?

    A   Frontal lobe
    B   Occipital lobe
    C   Parietal lobe
    D   Pituitary gland
    E   Temporal lobe

89. A 31-year-old man was diagnosed with Geschwind's syndrome. Which of the following statements is correct?

    A   It is a form of epilepsy.
    B   It is a personality syndrome encountered in subacute sclerosing panencephalitis.
    C   It is characterised by hypographia.
    D   It is characterised by hyposexuality.
    E   It is characterised by mutism.

90. A 39-year-old woman with irritable bowel syndrome (IBS) attended your clinic for an assessment. She would like to learn more about her condition. Which of the following statements about IBS is correct?

    A   Constipation-predominant group demonstrates abnormal adrenergic function.
    B   Constipation-predominant group has higher anxiety and depression rates.
    C   Diarrhoea-predominant group has higher anxiety and depression rates
    D   Diarrhoea-predominant group has vagal cholinergic function abnormalities.
    E   Patients with two gastrointestinal symptoms have lower rates of major depression than patients with one gastrointestinal symptom.

91. Which of the following statements about body mass index (BMI) is correct?

    A   A graded increase in schizophrenia is seen with increasing maternal BMI.
    B   A threefold increase in schizophrenia is seen in maternal BMI <17.5.
    C   It is defined as kilograms per centimetres squared.
    D   A low BMI is associated with neural tube defects.
    E   Normal range is between 17.5 and 28.

92. Group A β-haemolytic streptococci (GABHS) cause paediatric autoimmune neuropsychiatric disorders associated with streptococcal infections (PANDAS) consisting of five diagnostic criteria. Which of the following is a diagnostic criterion?

    A   Episodic course of symptom severity
    B   Insidious onset
    C   Postpubertal onset
    D   Presence of delirium
    E   Presence of panic attacks

93. A 37-year-old man with severe alcohol problems believed that his partner was unfaithful to him. He could not find any evidence but continued to hold his belief. What is the most likely diagnosis?

    A   Conjugal paranoia
    B   De Clérambault's syndrome
    C   Ekbom's syndrome
    D   Erotomania
    E   Folie-à-deux

94. Which of the following statements about *L'illusion des sosies* is correct?

    A   Geographical separation leads to recovery.
    B   It is a nihilistic delusional disorder.
    C   It is more common in women than in men.
    D   It is severe self-neglect seen in elderly people.
    E   Sufferers often lodge complaints and may engage in legal actions.

95. A 7-year-old boy refused to go to school and clung to his mother every time he was asked to get ready to go to school. His mother wanted to learn more about her son's condition. Which of the following statements about separation anxiety disorder is correct?

    A   About 10% of children and young adolescents have the disorder.
    B   Anxiety must last for a period of 6 weeks for a diagnosis to be made.
    C   In epidemiological studies, the disorder is more common in boys than girls.
    D   Onset of the disorder may occur any time before the age of 18.
    E   The disorder is unlikely to be exacerbated once it has remitted.

96. Which of the following pathological features of frontotemporal dementia is correct?

    A   Basal ganglia infarcts
    B   Deep white matter change
    C   Enlarged ventricles
    D   Generalised cerebral atrophy
    E   Knife-blade atrophy

97. Which of the following differentiates between ICD-10 and DSM-IV criteria for alcohol dependence?

    A   A strong desire or compulsion to use the substance
    B   Tolerance to the effects of the substance
    C   Continued use despite knowledge of harm
    D   Use of substance in larger quantities or longer than intended
    E   Withdrawal symptoms

98. A 45-year-old man, recently admitted to the ward for alcohol detoxification, started experiencing seizures. The seizures did not show any signs of stopping within 5 min of the onset. What is the treatment of choice?

    A   Chlordiazepoxide
    B   Intravenous diazepam
    C   General anaesthesia
    D   Phenytoin sodium
    E   Sodium valproate

99. A 27-year-man patient was undergoing treatment for drug misuse. Which of the following is a known method used to provide an effective incentive as part of contingency management?

    A   Clinic privileges
    B   Family-based reinforcement
    C   Friends-based reinforcement
    D   Home-based reinforcement
    E   School-based reinforcement

100. A 16-year-old boy with bipolar affective disorder had a relapse into acute mania. He was taking lithium carbonate and sodium valproate. It was decided to increase the dose of sodium valproate. What sodium valproate level should be aimed for?

    A   50 mg/L
    B   75 mg/L

C   100 mg/L
D   125 mg/L
E   150 mg/L

101. A 40-year-old alcohol-dependent man was brought to A&E by someone who found him roaming aimlessly. Which of the following features excludes Wernicke's encephalopathy?

    A   He was not oriented to time or place.
    B   On examination, he had nystagmus and lateral orbital palsy.
    C   The man had a very unsteady gait.
    D   The pupils were bilaterally constricted and symmetrical.
    E   When asked he said that he did not remember how he had come to the hospital.

102. Which of the following is most commonly associated with obsessive–compulsive disorder in children?

    A   Attention deficit hyperactivity disorder (ADHD)
    B   Autism
    C   Conduct disorder
    D   Schizophrenia
    E   Tic disorder

103. A 3-year-old boy with childhood autism was brought to your clinic for assessment. His mother would like to learn more about her son's condition and the long-term implications. What is the peak age of onset of seizures in someone with autism?

    A   0–4 years
    B   4–9 years
    C   9–11 years
    D   11–14 years
    E   14–17 years

104. A 9-year-old girl was diagnosed with pica. Her mother wanted to learn more about her daughter's condition. Which of the following statements about pica is correct?

    A   During this period the child develops an aversion to food.
    B   For a diagnosis, the child should eat non-nutritive substances for more than 6 months.
    C   It comes to clinical attention because of vitamin and mineral deficiencies.
    D   It is more commonly seen in older children.
    E   The disorder may continue into adulthood.

105. A 17-year-old boy was diagnosed with Gilles de la Tourette's syndrome. His father wanted to learn more about his son's condition. Which of the following statements about Gilles de la Tourette's syndrome is correct?

    A   It affects girls twice as much as boys.
    B   Coprolalia is present in about 25% of sufferers.
    C   It presents with multiple vocal and one or more motor tics.
    D   Median age of onset for motor tics is 6–7 years.
    E   Onset of disorder in 15% cases is above the age of 18.

106. Which of the following statements about assessment scales for depression in children and adolescents is correct?

    A   Beck's Depression Inventory (BDI) is used in children and adolescents.
    B   Children's Depression Inventory (CDI) has self, parent and teacher report forms.
    C   Children's Depression Rating Scale (CDRS) has 27 items.
    D   Centre for Epidemiological Studies – Depression (CES-D) is used in children.
    E   Mood and Feelings Questionnaire (MFQ) has 27 items.

107. Which of the following statements about the strange situation experiment is correct?

    A   Almost a third of children have anxious–avoidant attachment styles.
    B   Almost three-quarters of children are found to be securely attached.
    C   It was devised by Ainsworth and Wittig in 1869.
    D   Four types of attachment behaviours were identified from the experiment.
    E   The baby treats the stranger and the mother in the same way in an anxious–resistant type of attachment.

108. Which of the following is a parental vulnerability factor to be considered in identifying children at risk of developing conduct problems?

    A   All mothers are younger than 18 years
    B   At least one of the parents is on social security benefits
    C   At least one parent has a history of some contact with the criminal justice system
    D   Parents with education status below GCSE level
    E   Parents with other mental health problems

109. You were asked to see a 12-year-old boy with epilepsy and poor scholastic performance in school. He had an IQ assessment, which showed an IQ of 45. Which of the following categories describes his condition?

    A   Borderline learning disability
    B   Mild learning disability
    C   Moderate learning disability
    D   Profound learning disability
    E   Severe learning disability

110. An 8-year-old girl was diagnosed with nocturnal enuresis. Her mother wanted to learn more about the daughter's condition. Which of the following statements about enuresis is correct?

    A   Approximately 25% of children with the disorder have first-degree biological relatives with the disorder.
    B   Around 1% of adolescents aged >15 years have the disorder.
    C   Enuresis is repeated voiding of urine during the night into the bed or clothes.
    D   For a diagnosis, the chronological and mental age of the child must be ≥7 years.
    E   It is never an intentional act

111. Which of the following scales is useful in assessing disability in a learning-disabled population?

    A   Bender's gestalt test
    B   Raven's progressive matrices
    C   Vineland's Social Adaptive Behaviour Test
    D   Wechsler Adult Intelligence Scale
    E   Wechsler Intelligence Scale for Children

112. Which of the following conditions is detected using Guthrie's test?

    A   Coffin–Lowry syndrome
    B   Hunter's syndrome
    C   Lesch–Nyhan syndrome
    D   MASA syndrome
    E   Phenylketonuria

113. A 23-year-old man was recently diagnosed with schizophrenia. He attended your outpatient clinic for a review and was keen to know more about his condition. Which of the following is considered to be suggestive of a relatively poor prognosis in schizophrenia?

    A   Acute onset
    B   Family history of mood disorder

C   Florid delusions and hallucinations
D   Obvious precipitating factors
E   Onset at young age

114. A 15-year-old boy attended your clinic for a review. He had been exhibiting antisocial and aggressive behaviour over the past 2 years. His mother was concerned about the change in his behaviour. Which of the following statements about aggressive and self-injurious behaviour among people with learning disability is correct?

A   Learned aggression is uncommon among people with learning disability.
B   Self-injurious behaviour is more common in mild than moderate learning disability.
C   Self-injurious behaviour peaks between 15 and 20 years of age.
D   They are rarely an indication of psychiatric disorder.
E   They are unrelated to genetics contribution.

115. Which of the following patterns of psychopathology and maladaptive features is associated with fragile X syndrome?

A   Anxiety, fears, phobias, inattention, hyperactivity, social disinhibition, indiscriminate relating
B   Hyperphagia, non-food obsessions and compulsions, skin picking, temper tantrums, lability, under-activity
C   Infantile cat-like cry, hyperactivity, inattention, stereotypies, self-injury
D   Non-compliance, stubbornness, inattention, overactivity, argumentative, depression and dementia in adulthood
E   Social anxiety, shyness, gaze aversion, autism, inattention, hyperactivity, depression

116. Which of the following is a classified childhood disorder in DSM-IV?

A   Articulation disorder
B   Comprehension disorder
C   Mathematics disorder
D   Mixed phonological disorder
E   Writing disorder

117. During a hostage incident, a 25-year-old female hostage began to develop positive feelings towards her male captor. After her release, she sets up a fund to pay for his legal defence. Which of the following is a term describing this behaviour?

A   Denial
B   Learned helplessness
C   Stockholm syndrome
D   Patty Hearst
E   Resilience

118. A 3-year-old boy was diagnosed with childhood autism. He was not yet able to speak. His parents were keen to know the likelihood of him developing useful speech. Which of the following would be an appropriate response?

A   10%
B   30%
C   50%
D   70%
E   90%

119. Which of the following is a reported pre-condition for the development of Stockholm syndrome?

A   A short and emotionally charged event
B   An adverse environment shared by captors and captives

C   Lack of opportunities for a bond to develop
D   When hostages are 'dehumanised'
E   When threats to life are fulfilled

120. Which of the following statements about the HCR-20 is correct?

   A   It can be used in an actuarial manner.
   B   It can accurately predict risk of violence.
   C   It consists of five historical factors and ten clinical factors.
   D   Negative attitudes to health services are a risk management item.
   E   Psychopathy is a clinical factor.

121. Which of the following statements about the Sex Offender Treatment Programme (SOTP) therapy is correct?

   A   A major part of it is medication based.
   B   It can be done only in prisons.
   C   It is based on cognitive–behavioural theory.
   D   It is used only for people with mental illness.
   E   It is usually done as an individual therapy.

122. Which of the following statements about psychological intervention in children and young people who abuse alcohol is correct?

   A   Brief strategic family should be offered twice weekly for a month to support the family.
   B   Functional family therapy helps to focus on parents' wellbeing and parenting skills.
   C   Functional family therapy should be conducted over 6–9 months.
   D   Multidimensional family therapy should consist of 12–15 weekly sessions.
   E   Multidimensional family therapy should be offered over a period of 1 year.

123. Which of the following statements about psychiatric disorders in prisoners is correct?

   A   Depression and schizophrenia are the most common diagnoses.
   B   High rates of psychotic disorder exist in prisoners remanded for psychiatric reports.
   C   In sentenced prisoners, the prevalence of psychotic disorder is much higher than in the general population.
   D   Psychiatric symptoms are most common after 6 months of imprisonment.
   E   Under 10% have ICD-10-classifiable psychiatric disorder.

124. Which of the following is a contraindication for disulfiram treatment?

   A   Asthma
   B   Female gender
   C   Kidney disease
   D   Long-term heavy drinking
   E   Pre-existing heart disease

125. Which of the following is a class B drug?

   A   Amphetamine, if snorted
   B   Cocaine, if injected
   C   Cocaine, if snorted
   D   Crack cocaine, if smoked
   E   MDMA

126. Which of the following statements about British law pertaining to cannabis is correct?

   A   An adult in possession will usually be arrested each time.
   B   It was reclassified from class B to class A in 2009.

C The maximum penalty for possession of cannabis is 6 months.
D The maximum penalty for supplying, producing and trafficking is 2 years of imprisonment.
E Young people in possession will receive a reprimand, final warning or charge if caught for the first time.

127. An 18-year-old female student was referred by her GP to mental health services because of extreme anxiety over the shape of her nose. Which of the following statements about dysmorphophobia (body dysmorphic disorder) is correct?

A It is classified as a hypochondriacal disorder in the ICD-10.
B It is more common in married patients than in those who are single.
C It is uncommon to have an underlying personality disorder.
D It usually takes the form of a delusional belief.
E There is usually no defect in appearance.

128. Limb pain, Brown–Séquard paralysis, multiple sclerosis, hypochondriasis, depersonalisation disorder, conversion disorder and anorexia nervosa share some common symptoms. Which of the following occurs in all of the above conditions?

A Asyndesis
B Hyperschemazia
C Kinaesthetic hallucinations
D Metamorphosis
E Phantom limb

129. Which of the following is an empirically supported treatment for adults with multiple mental health problems at risk of suicide?

A Cognitive–behavioural therapy
B Dialectical behaviour therapy
C Fluoxetine
D Systemic family therapy
E Venlafaxine

130. Which of the following is the most appropriate indication for experimental studies?

A Gold standard for establishing treatment efficacy
B One in which associations can be established but not the causation
C Suitable for a rare disease
D Suitable for a rare exposure
E Suitable to find out the prognosis

Questions: EMIs

Theme: Neuropsychiatric disorders in old age

Options for questions: 131–135

A   Cortical dementia
B   Delusional disorder
C   Dementia-related psychosis
D   Extradural haemorrhage
E   Hyperactive delirium
F   Hypoactive delirium
G   Late-onset schizophrenia
H   Lewy body dementia
I   Subcortical dementia
J   Subdural haematoma

For each of the following cases, select the single most appropriate diagnosis. Each option may be used once, more than once or not at all.

131. A 65-year-old woman has had REM sleep behaviour disorder for 10 years. She has had conversations with her deceased loved ones and experienced visual hallucinations. Her condition deteriorated after she was given an antiemetic for severe dyspepsia.

132. An 80-year-old woman with hepatitis presented with acute confusion, depressed level of consciousness, lethargy and sluggishness.

133. A 40-year-old female cricketer was hit on her head by a cricket ball in a friendly match. She lost consciousness for a few seconds but regained it and started playing again. When the match ended, she became extremely delirious with laboured breathing.

134. A 70-year-old woman has developed problems with her language, judgement, memory, problem-solving and reasoning over the past couple of years.

135. A 72-year-old, socially isolated, elderly woman with some hearing problems attended her GP and elaborated on a systematised persecutory delusional system involving threat to her home.

Theme: Comparison of relationships between different variables

Options for questions: 136–140

A   Correlation coefficient
B   Kendall's correlational coefficient
C   Logistic regression
D   Multiple analysis of covariance
E   Multiple analysis of variance
F   Multiple linear regression
G   Pearson's correlational coefficient
H   Proportional Cox's regression
I   Simple linear regression
J   Spearman's rank correlation coefficient

For each of the following cases, select the single most appropriate response. Each option may be used once, more than once or not at all.

136. It is used for predicting the dependent variable from two or more independent variables.

137. It is a correlational coefficient for two normally distributed variables.

138. It is used to assess survival or other time-related events.

139. Where there are two variables, one independent (X) and one dependent (Y), i.e. change in X causes a change in Y.

140. It is a correlational coefficient in which one variable is normally distributed and the other is categorical or non-normally distributed.

Theme: Types of data and distribution

Options for questions: 141–143

A   Continuous distribution
B   Discrete data
C   Gaussian distribution
D   Nominal data
E   Negatively skewed distribution
F   Ordinal data
G   Positively skewed distribution
H   Uniform distribution

For each of the following cases, select the single most appropriate distribution. Each option may be used once, more than once or not at all.

141. In a study of depression you obtain data on the gender of each participant

142. The measurement of body weight in a study of adolescent anorexia patients

143. You decided to do a patient satisfaction survey measuring it on a 5-point scale of not satisfied to very satisfied

Theme: Risk of developing a psychiatric disorder

Options for questions: 144–146

A   3%
B   8%
C   15%
D   25%
E   46%
F   55%
G   70%
H   85%

For each of the following cases, select the single most appropriate figure. Each option may be used once, more than once or not at all.

144. A 28-year-old woman was under your care for schizophrenia. Her 32-year-old partner also had a history of schizophrenia. The illness of both patients has been under good control for the last 2–3 years. She wishes to start a family and wants to know the likelihood of their child developing schizophrenia.

145. A 35-year-old woman with bipolar affective disorder wanted to start a family. She was worried about the risk of developing puerperal psychosis after her delivery because her mother had a similar history. She wanted to know the likelihood of having an episode of postpartum psychosis.

146. The mother of a 22-year-old man with schizophrenia was worried about her younger son developing the same illness. He is 14 years old. She wanted to know the likelihood of her younger son developing schizophrenia.

Theme: Culture-bound syndrome

Options for questions: 147–149

A   Amok
B   Ataque de nervios
C   Bouffée délirante
D   Brain fag
E   Dhat
F   Koro
G   Latah
H   Piblokto
I   Susto
J   Zar

For each of the following cases, select the single most appropriate diagnosis. Each option may be used once, more than once or not at all.

147. A 35-year-old Puerto Rican man, following his wife's unexpected death, went into a trance-like state with unpredictable behaviour. He recovered after a few days but had no recollection of his condition.

148. A 27-year-old West African man complained of a variety of psychosomatic symptoms that he attributed to overwork, tiredness and 'too much thinking'. He complained of reduced concentration.

149. A 35-year-old single Malaysian man believed that his genitals were retracting into his abdomen and, once this happened, he would die immediately.

Theme: Mechanism of action for drugs used in the treatment of dementia

Options for questions: 150–152

A	Acetylcholine receptor modulation	F	NMDA antagonist
B	Butyrylcholinesterase inhibition	G	NMDA-receptor agonist
C	Choline Inhibitor	H	Non-competitive inhibition of acetylcholinesterase
D	Competitive inhibition of acetylcholinesterase	I	Nootropic properties
E	Nicotinic receptor modulation		

For each of the following drugs, select the most appropriate mechanism of action according to further instruction. Each option may be used once, more than once or not at all.

150. Donepezil [select ONE option]

151. Galantamine [select TWO options]

152. Memantine [select ONE option]

Theme: Risk assessment in elderly people

Options for questions: 153–155

A	Aggression	F	Flooding
B	Emotional abuse	G	Self-harm
C	Falls	H	Self-neglect
D	Financial abuse	I	Wandering
E	Fire		

For each of the following cases, select the most appropriate risk factors according to further instruction. Each option may be used once, more than once or not at all.

153. A 68-year-old woman stopped going out, eating and drinking. She had lost 10 kg in weight. She believed that she had a terminal illness and was going to die [select TWO options].

154. An 82-year-old man with vascular dementia had become more agitated and confused. He had been resisting the care given by the staff. He lived in a care home [select THREE options].

155. A 74-year-old man with vascular dementia appeared to have had a further TIA, with increasingly unsteady gait [select ONE option].

Theme: Intoxication symptoms due to chemical substances

Options for questions: 156–158

A	Alcohol	E	Heroin
B	Amphetamines	F	Inhalants
C	Cannabis	G	LSD
D	Cocaine	H	Nicotine

For each of the following cases, select the single most appropriate drug. Each option may be used once, more than once or not at all.

156. A 19-year-old university student presented with marked anxiety, severe restlessness, hallucinations and confusion. His friends said that he had been stressed lately because of the exams and was staying up till the early hours of the morning cramming.

157. A 30-year-old man with depression was brought to A&E by the police. On examination, his speech was slurred, he was drowsy and his pupils were constricted. There were multiple bruises on his arms.

158. A 19-year-old man known to the early intervention-in-psychosis team presented with an inappropriately euphoric mood after a weekend trip with his friends. On examination, he showed impaired coordination, tachycardia and conjunctival injection. He described seeing vivid colours and claimed to have a special knowledge of time.

Theme: Prevalence of illnesses in children and adolescents

Options for questions: 159–161

A	Attention deficit hyperactivity disorder (ADHD)	E	Encopresis in 5 year olds
B	Anxiety disorders	F	Enuresis in 5-year-old children
C	Developmental coordination disorder	G	Major depression in children
D	Dysthymia	H	Selective mutism
		I	Separation anxiety disorder

For each of the following figures, select the single most appropriate diagnosis. Each option may be used once, more than once or not at all.

159 <1%

160. 5%

161. 5–10%

Theme: Assessment tools used in forensic services

Options for questions: 162–166

A	Historical, Clinical, Risk Management 20 (HCR-20)	E	Psychopathy Check List – Revised (PCL-R)
		F	Risk of Sexual Violence Protocol (RSVP)
B	International Personality Disorder Examination (IPDE)	G	Sexual Offending Risk Appraisal Guide (SORAG)
C	Matrix 2000	H	Spousal Assault Risk Assessment (SARA)
D	Millon Clinical Multi-axial Inventory (MCMI)	I	Violence Risk Appraisal Guide (VRAG)

For each of the following cases, select the most appropriate assessment tool (s) according to further instructions. Each option may be used once, more than once or not at all.

162. A 35-year-old man convicted of a rape offence was given a secure hospital disposal. The clinical team would like to use a structured clinical judgement tool to formulate the risk of sexual offending]select ONE option].

163. A 22-year-old man was convicted of murder. He had a long history of violence which did not result in convictions in the past. His assessments noted the following traits: lack of empathy, repeated lying, manipulation, glibness and a lack of remorse [select TWO options].

164. A 30-year-old woman was admitted to a secure hospital for assessment after an arson offence. The treating team had given her a self-report questionnaire to assess her premorbid personality [select ONE option].

165. A probation officer would like to assess the violence risk for a 30-year-old community patient who has assaulted his wife. She had requested an actuarial assessment tool [select ONE option].

166. An offender manager would like to assess the risk of sexual offending by a 52-year-old male inmate before his parole hearing. He would like an actuarial assessment of risk [select TWO options].

Theme: Chromosomal abnormalities associated with learning difficulties

Options for questions: 167–171

A   Angelman's syndrome
B   Cri-du-chat syndrome
C   DiGeorge's (velocardiofacial) syndrome
D   Edwards' syndrome
E   Fragile C syndrome
F   Prader–Willi syndrome
G   Smith–Magenis syndrome
H   Turner's syndrome
I   Williams' syndrome

For each of the following cases, select the single most appropriate diagnosis. Each option may be used once, more than once or not at all.

167. 15q12 deletion, maternally inherited

168. 17q deletion

168. Trisomy 18

170. 22q11.2

171. 7q11.2

Theme: Randomisation methods in research studies

Options for questions: 172–175

A   Minimisation
B   Play the winner
C   Simple randomisation
D   Stratified randomisation
E   Randomised consent method
F   Randomisation permutated blocks

For each of the following cases, select the single most appropriate randomisation method. Each option may be used once, more than once or not at all.

172. In this method, the first participant is allocated by a simple randomisation procedure and then after every subsequent allocation it is based on the success or failure of the immediate predecessor participant.

173. This technique is useful for studies of small size and long duration in which it can ensure that roughly comparable numbers of participants are allocated to study groups at any point in the process.

174. In this method, an eligible population is divided according to a minimum number of important prognostic factors.

175. This method is used in some clinical trials to lessen the effect of some patients refusing to participate.

Theme: Design features of clinical research studies

Options for questions: 176–178

A   Control participants receive a placebo
B   Each group receives a different treatment with both groups being entered at the same time
C   Each participant received both the intervention and the treatment
D   Participants are assessed before and after an intervention
E   Results are analysed by comparing groups
F   Results are analysed in terms of differences between participant pairs
G   Separated by a period of no treatment
H   This permits an investigation of the effects of more than one independent variable on a given outcome

For each of the following studies, select TWO most appropriate features. Each option may be used once, more than once or not at all.

176. Cross-over trial

177. Parallel-group comparison

178. Paired comparison

Theme: Randomised control trials

Options for questions: 179–181

A   Assumes a poor outcome for drop-outs
B   'Brought forward' data are incorporated into the overall analysis of whichever group they originally belonged to
C   Data should be analysed as a unit of randomisation
D   Data on all patients entering a trial should be analysed with respect to the groups to which they were originally randomised, regardless of whether or not they received treatment
E   Differences in the drop-out rates and the timing of these drop-outs influence the estimation of treatment
F   Interventions are directed at groups rather than individual participants
G   This may not be appropriate in trials assessing the physiological effects of a drug as opposed to efficacy

For each of the following descriptions, select TWO most appropriate options. Each option may be used once, more than once or not at all.

179. Last data carried forward

180. Intention-to-treat analysis

181. Cluster trials

Theme: Costs involved in healthcare

Options for questions: 182–184

A   Avoiding hospital admission
B   Investigations
C   Pain and suffering
D   Prevention of expensive-to-treat illness
E   Social stigma
F   Staff salaries
H   Value of 'unpaid work'
I   Work days lost

For each of the following descriptions, select the TWO most appropriate cost options. Each option may be used once, more than once or not at all.

182. Direct costs

183. Intangible costs

184. Indirect costs

Theme: Medical databases

Options for questions: 185–187

A Allied and Complementary Medicine Database (AMED)
B Cumulative Index to Nursing and Allied Health Literature (CINAHL)
C Cochrane Library
D EMBASE
E Google Scholar
F Health STAR
G MEDLINE
H PsycINFO
I Scopus

For each of the following descriptions, select the single most appropriate database. Each option may be used once, more than once or not at all.

185. It covers health services, hospital administration and health technology assessment.

186. This is a nursing and allied health database.

187. The database of Excerpta Medica focuses on drugs and pharmacology, clinical medicine and other biomedical specialties.

Theme: Architecture of clinical research

Options for questions: 188–190

A Causation can be inferred
B Examples include controlled clinical trial and economic analyses, systematic reviews and their meta-analyses
C Examples include case-control and cohort studies
D Examples include case reports and series, audits, cross-sectional surveys and qualitative study
E Generally compare two groups
F Generally conducted without a control group
G Something is given or done in the experimental group but not in the control group
H Suitable for hypothesis generation
I Suitable for hypothesis testing

For each of the following studies, select THREE most appropriate descriptions. Each option may be used once, more than once or not at all.

188. Descriptive studies

189. Analytical studies

190. Experimental studies

Theme: Sources of bias in clinical drug trials

Options for questions: 191–194

A Double blinding
B Information bias
C Observer bias
D Recall bias

E   Selection bias
F   Single blinding
G   Triple blinding

For each of the following descriptions, select the single most appropriate source of bias. Each option may be used once, more than once or not at all.

191. It reduces the potential bias of a patient's placebo response.

192. It reduces the doctor's sometimes overzealous desire to find a good new treatment.

193. The analysis of outcomes is conducted by an independent researcher.

194. This is prone to non-blind outcome assessment.

Theme: Measures of disease frequency

Options for questions: 195–198

A   Incidence density
B   Incidence risk
C   Lifetime risk
D   Mortality ratio
E   Period prevalence
F   Point prevalence
G   Standardised mortality ratio

For each of the following cases, select the single most appropriate option. Each option may be used once, more than once or not at all.

195. The number of new cases of the disease over a period of time out of the total population at risk.

196. The number of new cases out of the person-time of observation.

197. The number of individuals with the disease in the population over a period of time.

198. The ratio of observed to expected deaths.

Theme: Neurological symptoms after head injury

Options for questions: 199 and 200

A   Dysphasia
B   Dysprosody
C   Jargon aphasia
D   Post-concussion syndrome
E   Reduplicative paramnesia
F   Visual agnosia

For each of the following cases, select the single most appropriate diagnosis. Each option may be used once, more than once or not at all.

199. Any delusion involving duplication, e.g. that events have been duplicated or that the patient has a second left leg.

200. A phenomenon in which the normal rhythms and intonations of speech are lost.

Answers: MCQs

1. D Delusional perception

This refers to the attribution of a new meaning, usually in the sense of self-reference to a normally perceived object. The new meaning cannot be understood as arriving from the patient's affective state or previous attitudes. The latter proviso is important because the delusional perception must not be confused with delusional misinterpretation. Schneider emphasised the importance of this symptom's 'two memberedness' because there is a link between a real perception and a new meaning attached to the perception. It is a primary delusion (also called apophany or autochthonous delusion) and is diagnostic of schizophrenia. Delusional mood refers to the condition when the patient knows that there is something going on around him that concerns him but he does understand what it is. Delusional memory consists of two parts: the perception (either real or imagined) and the memory. It is defined differently by some authorities, e.g. a delusional interpretation of real memories or an experience of past events that did not occur, but the patient remembers that they did indeed occur. Delusional misinterpretation refers to attribution of meaning to a normal perception as a result of a pre-existing delusion.

2. A Oxygen is administered before ECT

Following ECT treatment patients have to wait in the recovery area until they regain full consciousness and have no complications. The referring psychiatrist can prescribe two sessions at a time, after which the patient has to be reviewed before a further prescription of ECT is given. Routinely, up to two ECT sessions are given in 1 week. ECT-induced seizures are generalised tonic clonic seizures.

3. B Rare exposures

The cohort study is suitable for rare exposures and multiple outcomes. It is unsuitable for rare diseases. It is usually a prospective epidemiological study of one or more groups, which are defined by the presence or absence of an exposure, i.e. aetiology, or disease, i.e. outcome. It does not necessarily need a control group. The cohort study can be conducted retrospectively when the cohort has already been exposed and possibly developed the disease. It is less liable to bias than other observational studies, especially recall bias and reverse causality. However, participants lost to follow-up will affect the validity.

4. D Reflex hallucination

A stimulus in one sensory modality producing a hallucination in another is called a reflex hallucination. This is a morbid form of synaesthesia, which is the experience of a stimulus image in one modality producing an image in another, e.g. a man felt a pain in his head (somatic hallucination) when he heard other people shouting (the stimulus) and became convinced that the shouting caused the pain in head. Autoscopy refers to phantom mirror image, which is the experience of seeing oneself and knowing that it is oneself. It is clearly not a pure visual hallucination because kinaesthetic and somatic perception must be present to experience mirror image. It is also called the doppelganger phenomenon. Autoscopy can occur in healthy people, psychotic disorders, organic conditions, e.g. epilepsy, toxic infective states, parieto-occipital lesions, and as a hysterical symptom. A functional hallucination requires the presence of another real stimulus to experience a hallucination in the same modality. An extracampine hallucination refers to a hallucination that is outside the limits of the sensory field.

5. E Stem-and-leaf plot

This is also called a 'stem plot'. It is a method for demonstrating the frequency with which certain classes of values occur, and is also used to present quantitative data in a graphical format. The 'stem' values are listed down and the 'leaf' values go to the right or left of the stem values. The 'stem' is used to group the scores and each 'leaf' indicates the individual scores within each group. For a stem plot, the statistical data are preferably arranged in ascending order because it is basically plotting the statistical data as per the individual place value. The number on the left (e.g. 1 is the 'left' number in 10, the tenth place or tens) is considered to be the 'stem' and the numbers on the right (0 is the 'right' number in 10, the one place or units) of each data item are plotted as 'leaves'.

A histogram looks similar to a bar chart with no gaps between adjacent bars. It is used with metric continuous data and the data are grouped together before being plotted on the histogram. In a dot plot for continuous data, a dot is placed in for each observation along one axis. The scatter plot helps in evaluating the association between two variables. The box-and-whisker plot has a rectangle that extends from the end of the first quartile to the start of the fourth quartile of observations. The whiskers show the upper and lower limits. The median value is represented by a line transecting the rectangle.

6. E Thomas Szaz

All of the people (except Freud) mentioned in the question were associated with the anti-psychiatry movement. Most notably, Thomas Szaz wrote Myth of Mental Illness. Goffman's main contribution to psychiatry was his work on institutionalisation of psychiatric patients. Foucault wrote Madness and Civilization: A history of insanity in the age of reason. RD Laing wrote several books including The Divided Self: An existential study in sanity and madness, Sanity and Madness in the Family, The Facts of Life and Politics of Experience.

7. B Cost-effectiveness analysis

This is used when the effect of the interventions can be expressed in terms of one main variable. The outcome measures are natural units, e.g. life-years saved. The cost-minimisation analysis is used when the effect of both interventions is known. The cost–utility analysis is used when the effect of the intervention has two or more important dimensions. The outcome could be quality-adjusted life-years (QALYs). The cost–benefit analysis is used to compare the intervention for one condition with an intervention for a different condition. It compares the costs and outcomes of two or more therapeutic interventions in terms of monetary cost. The fiscal impact analysis is used by the government to study the revenue, expenditure and savings that will result from the proposed policy or programme.

8. A Cyproterone acetate causes side effects similar to those of surgical castration.

Due to its anti-androgenic and progestogenic action, cyproterone acetate causes a reduction in the levels of testosterone, FSH (follicle-stimulating hormone) and LH (luteinising hormone), and increase the levels of serum prolactin. By blocking the testosterone receptors, cyproterone acetate leads to 'chemical castration' and the effects are as good as surgical castration. Its main therapeutic indications include prostate cancer, benign prostatic hypertrophy, priapism and hypersexuality. It can be used to treat acne and hirsutism in women and as hormone therapy in male-to-female transsexuals. It inhibits spermatogenesis and produces reversible infertility.

9. E Protocol for storing of Dantrolene should be available

ECTAS specifies there is a requirement to have a separate protocol for maintenance treatment for ECT, treatment for young people under 18 years and those with malignant hyperthermia. Policies relating to ECT must be checked once every 2 years.

10. E 15.33

Likelihood ratio of a positive test (LR+) = Sensitivity/(1 − Specificity)

= 0.92/(1 − 0.94)

= 15.33.

The likelihood ratio is the value of a given test that results in prediction of the presence of a disease.

11. B Feeling punished

Somatic symptoms of depression such as weight loss, sleep disturbance, lethargy and psychomotor retardation can at times be due to physical illness. Cognitive symptoms help to differentiate depressed from non-depressed patients. Three main affective symptoms have been described such as depressed mood, hopelessness and helplessness, which can help the differentiation. In addition, patients may feel punished, and have inappropriate guilt, poor self-esteem and suicidal ideation.

12. D Sertraline

This is the first choice for depression in patients who have had a myocardial infarction. However, if possible, all antidepressants should be avoided for the first 2 months after a myocardial infarction, although they are not contraindicated. Dothiepin can cause a dose-related increase in ischaemic heart disease when compared with patients who have never taken dothiepin. Venlafaxine is known to cause hypertension. Lithium can cause changes in the ECG such as wide QRS complexes, or flat or inverted T waves. It is used with caution if needed. There is insufficient evidence for the use of agomelatine in patients who have had a myocardial infarction.

13. E 0.88

The positive predictive value (PPV) is the proportion of people with a positive test result who actually have the illness. It is also called a precision rate. It is therefore the proportion of participants with positive test results who are true positives. Positive and negative predictive values, sensitivity and specificity are related.

PPV = $a/(a + b)$

= 80/(80 + 10) = 0.88 (88%).

14. C 0.77

The negative predictive value (NPV) is the proportion of participants with a negative test result who were correctly diagnosed, i.e. they actually do not have the disease.

NPV = $d/(c + d)$

= 70/(70 + 20) = 0.77 (77%).

15. C 6.15

LR+ = Sensitivity/(1 − Specificity)

The sensitivity is the proportion of people with the illness who have a positive result:

Sensitivity = $a/(a + c)$

= 80/100 = 0.80 (80%).

The specificity is the proportion of people without the illness who have a negative test = $d/(b +d)$:

Specificity = 70/80 = 0.87 (87%).

LR+ = 0.80/(1 − 0.87)

= 0.80/0.13 = 6.15.

16. B 0.22

LR− = (1 − Sensitivity)/Specificity

= (1 − 0.8)/0.87

= 0.22.

Important formulae and definitions

The people who have a disorder and a positive test are called true positives. The proportion of the people with the disorder who have a positive test is called the sensitivity of the test:

Sensitivity = $a/(a + c)$.

The people who do not have the disorder and have a negative test are called true negatives:

Specificity = $d/(b + d)$.

In a screening test, the positive predictive value (PPV) is the proportion of people with a positive test who have the illness:

PPV = $a/(a + b)$.

In a screening test, the negative predictive value (NPV) is the proportion of people with a negative test who do not have the illness:

NPV = $d/(c + d)$.

The likelihood ratio for a positive test (LR+) result is the value that result has in predicting the presence of the disorder. It is usually >1.

LR+ = Sensitivity/(1 − Specificity).

The likelihood ratio for a negative test (LR−) is the probability of a negative test in those with the disorder divided by the probability of a negative test in those without the disorder. It is usually <1.

LR− = (1 − Sensitivity)/Specificity.

17. D HIV-associated dementia

HIV-associated dementia is the most common CNS complication of HIV disease and generally carries a poor prognosis. It acts by direct invasion of the brain by HIV. Around 60% of patients dying of HIV show some degree of dementia. Direct HIV-associated pathology of the CNS includes

HIV encephalitis, HIV leukoencephalopathy, vacuolar myelopathy (spinal cord infection), vacuolar leukoencephalopathy, diffuse poliodystrophy, cerebral vasculitis, including granulomatous angiitis, and lymphocytic meningitis. There is substantial neuronal loss, with around 38% depletion of neurons, especially in the frontal lobes. There is a significant association between such neuronal loss and dementia.

18. D Paranoid personality disorder

People with high levels of paranoid thinking have an externalising personal attributional bias, which is a tendency to explain negative events in their life by blaming others rather than reflecting on their own potential contribution to the circumstances. In paranoid personality disorder, the normal self-serving bias, whereby negative events are attributed to external circumstances, is exaggerated and distorted, it being skewed towards other people's malevolent intent.

19. E The primary outcome measure was quality of life.

In the Cost Utility of the Latest Antipsychotic Drugs in Schizophrenia 1 (CUtLASS 1) study, the main outcome measures were scores on quality-of-life scales, symptoms, adverse effects, participant satisfaction and care costs. The patients on first-generation antipsychotics showed greater improvement in the quality-of-life scales and symptom scores. Compared with the atypical (second-generation) antipsychotics, the conventional (first-generation) antipsychotics were more cost-effective (>50%) and had more QALYs.

20. E Victims are often not believed by others.

A previous partner who takes on a stalking behaviour represents a significant risk. Victims are often subjected to a range of stalking behaviour and harassment, often for long periods of time. These victims are more likely to be physically assaulted. Recovery from these experiences is often complicated by feelings of guilt and self-blame. The impact of stalking depends on the victim's characteristics, past experience, knowledge of the stalker and the present circumstances. There is a wide range of effects on the victim's mental and physical health, social life, work and finances. Male victims experience symptoms similar to those reported by female victims.

21. E <1:5000

The risk of agranulocytosis with clozapine treatment in the UK is <1:5000. It is a serious, life-threatening, adverse effect of clozapine. Almost 0.8% of clozapine-treated patients develop potentially fatal agranulocytosis, with the risk being highest within the first 18 weeks of treatment. The risk of death from agranulocytosis is probably <1:10 000 patients taking clozapine. Increasing age and Asian race are major risk factors. Lithium does not protect against clozapine-induced agranulocytosis. This risk is managed by clozapine monitoring systems in the UK and other countries.

Answers: MCQs

22. A Confabulation

Table 3.3 Distortions of recall

Retrospective falsification	Unintentional distortion of memory that occurs when it is filtered through a person's current emotional, experiential and cognitive state
False memory	Recollection of an event that did not occur but that the individual subsequently strongly believes did take place
Screen memory	Recollection that is partially true and partially false. It is thought that the individual recalls only part of the true memory because the entirety of the true memory is too painful to recall
Confabulation	Falsification of memory occurring in clear consciousness in association with organic pathology. It manifests itself as the filling in of gaps in memory by imagined or untrue experiences that have no basis in fact
Pseudologica fantastica	Fluent plausible lying. Used to describe the confabulation that occurs in those without organic brain pathology such as personality disorder of antisocial or hysterical type
Munchausen's syndrome	Variant of pathological lying in which the individual presents to hospitals with bogus illnesses, complex medical histories and often multiple surgical scars
Vorbeireden	Approximate answers, seen in those with hysterical pseudo-dementia
Cryptamnesia	'The experience of not remembering that one is remembering'
Retrospective delusions	Found in some patients with psychoses who backdate their delusions in spite of clear evidence that the illness is of recent origin

23. E 1:4500

There is a possible association between clozapine and thromboembolism. A study reported a risk of fatal pulmonary embolism of 1 in 4500 clozapine patients, which is about 20 times the risk in the population as a whole. It is most likely to occur in the first 3 months of treatment but can occur at any time. Its causes are multifactorial, but it is thought to be related to clozapine's effects on anti-phospholipid antibodies and platelet aggregation. The essential preventive measures include regular exercise and good hydration.

24. B Sertraline

In patients with renal impairment, one should choose a drug cautiously and avoid drugs that are nephrotoxic and extensively cleared by the kidneys. The dosage should be low to start with; it needs gradual titration and frequent monitoring. In the case of sertraline the dosing is as for a patient with normal renal function. However, sertraline is associated with acute renal failure and, therefore, should be used cautiously. The dosage needs adjustment, according to the estimated glomerular filtration rate (eGFR), for clomipramine, mirtazapine, reboxetine and venlafaxine.

25. D 90%

To calculate sensitivity, one can construct a 2 × 2 table with the gold standard results at the top. It is advisable to follow one style using columns and rows to indicate a particular group of data. Table 3.4 is drawn with the gold standard results across the two data columns, and screening questionnaire results across the rows.

Table 3.4 A 2 × 2 table

Depression identified by two-item screening questionnaire	ICD-10 diagnosis of depression		Total
	Yes	No	
Yes	45 (a)	50 (b)	95 (a + b)
No	5 (c)	85 (d)	90 (c + d)
Total	50 (a + c)	135 (b + d)	185 (a + b + c + d)

Sensitivity is defined as the test's ability to identify people who, according to the diagnostic gold standard, actually have the disorder, i.e. true positives. In other words, sensitivity is the proportion of time-positive (cases) correctly identified by the test:

Sensitivity = $a/(a + c)$ = (45/50) × 100 = 90%.

26. B 63%

Specificity is defined as the test's ability to exclude people who, according to the diagnostic (gold) standard, do not actually have the disorder, i.e. true negatives. It is the proportion of true negatives among all non-diseased individuals. In other words, it is the ability of a test to rule out the disorder among people who do not have it.

Specificity = $d/(b + d)$

= 85/(50 + 85) = (85/135) × 100

= 62.96 = 63%.

27. B 47%

It is understood that not all people who are found to be positive on the test might actually have the disorder. It is therefore necessary to work out how many people diagnosed with depression using the screening questionnaire actually have it. The power of a test is the likelihood or probability of the test rejecting the null hypothesis when it is incorrect. PPV gives the proportion of true positives among the test positives. It is calculated by using the formula:

PPV = $a/(a + b)$

= 45/(45 + 50) × 100 = 47%.

28. E 94%

It is understood that people who have been found to be 'negative' on the test might actually be disease free. The NPV answers the above matter. It is calculated by the formula:

NPV = $d/(c + d)$

= 85/(5 + 85) = (85/90) × 100 = 94%.

29. B. 0.16

The LR– is the likelihood that a negative test comes from a person without the disorder rather than someone with the disorder. To be useful in excluding the disorder, the LR- should be <1. If the ratio is 0, it will be perfect in predicting an absence of the disorder, but it will be of no value in predicting the presence of a disorder. It is determined by the probability of a negative test in people with the disorder divided by the probability of a negative disorder in those without the disorder. LR- is calculated by the formula:

LR– = (1 – Sensitivity)/Specificity

= [$c/(a + c)$]/[$d/(b + d)$]

= [5/(45+5)]/[85/(50+85)] = [(5/50)]/[(85/135)]

= 0.1/0.63 = 0.158.

30. C 27%

The pre-test probability is the same as the base rate or prevalence. It refers to the proportion of people who have the target disorder in a population at risk at a specific point or interval. It is calculated by the formula:

$(a + c)/n$ = (45 + 5)/185 = (50/185) × 100 = 27%

where n is the total population measured.

The post-test probability is the prevalence of the disorder in people with a positive test. It is a useful estimate of the PPV in these people.

31. C 37%

A false positive (FP) is a situation where a person is diagnosed with the new test as having a condition, when according to the gold standard he or she does not actually have it. In the given situation, it is the percentage of people falsely identified by the test as depressed. Using the 2 × 2 table, the false-positive rate is calculated by the formula:

FP = $b/(b + d)$ = 50/(50 + 35)

= (50/135) × 100 = 37%.

32. B 10%

A false negative (FN) is a situation in which a person is not diagnosed as having a condition with the new test when, according to the gold standard, he or she actually has it. In the given situation, it is the percentage of people among the depressed group who are falsely identified by the test as not depressed. The false-negative rate is calculated by the formula:

FN = $c/(a + c)$ = 5/(45 + 5)

= (5/50) × 100 = 10%.

33. E Progressive encephalopathy in children is due to primary HIV infection of the CNS.

There are four categories of infections in HIV:

1 Group 1 (acute infection): transient symptoms at the time or just after seroconversion

2 Group 2: asymptomatic infection
3 Group 3: persistent generalised lymphadenopathy (PGL) or lymphadenopathy syndrome (LAS)
4 Group 4: other diseases, i.e. AIDS-related complex and AIDS.

The nervous system is an early target in HIV infection. Neurological involvement starts very early in the disease and 90% of cases with AIDS will have neuropathological changes *post mortem*. Neuropsychiatric manifestations of CNS in HIV are due to:

- Opportunistic infections of the CNS: viral, fungal and parasitic infections are common. Bacterial infections are rare.
- Neoplasia of the CNS: the most common CNS neoplasm is primary non-Hodgkin's malignant lymphoma, occurring in around 2–6% of patients.
- Primary HIV infection of the CNS: the AIDS–dementia complex or HIV-associated dementia and progressive encephalopathy in children are due to primary HIV infection of the CNS.

34. B PLC is an essential part of the pseudo-bulbar palsy syndrome.

PLC is usually triggered by a stimulus that would not normally trigger the response of laughter or crying. It is frequent, brief and intense paroxysms of uncontrollable crying and/or laughing, mainly due to a neurological disorder. The Pathological Laughter and Crying Scale (PLACS) is useful for assessing the severity of symptoms in a pathological emotional display.

Bilateral lesions in the corticobulbar tracts may lead to pseudo-bulbar palsy, which in turn can cause PLC. There is altered emotional expression due to disruption of prefrontal regulation of the limbic circuits. PLC is often misunderstood and can be a cause of distress to patients and their families because it affects interpersonal functioning and/or activities of daily living. SSRIs are the first line of choice. Tricyclic antidepressants, non-competitive NMDA (N-methyl-d-aspartate) receptor antagonists, dopaminergic agents and noradrenergic reuptake inhibitors or novel antidepressants can be used if SSRIs are not successful. PLC is seen in almost 40%, 19–49%, 10–20% and 7–10% of patients with Alzheimer's disease, amyotrophic lateral sclerosis, stroke and multiple sclerosis, respectively.

35. C 15%

It should be noted that the prevalence of a condition can vary according to the population tested. The prevalence rate or pre-test probability of depression in the given population is 15%. To calculate the PPV of the two-item screening questionnaire, it is necessary to use 2 × 2 tables, and the sensitivity and specificity of the questionnaire for the disease. From the given information, the prevalence is $(a + c) \times n = 15\%$. The value of n is 1500, so $a + c = 100$.

Sensitivity = 90%:

$a/(a + c) = a/100 = 0.90$,

so $a = 90$.

Specificity = 63%:

$d/(b + d) = d/1400 = 0.63$,

so $d = 1400 \times 0.63 = 882$.

Once we know *a* and *d* the 2 × 2 table can be drawn (**Table 3.5**).

Table 3.5 A 2 × 2 table

Screening questionnaire	ICD-10 gold standard		
	Depression present	Depression absent	Total
Positive	90 (a)	518 (b)	608 (a + b)
Negative	10 (c)	882 (d)	892 (c + d)
Total	100 (a + c)	1400 (b + d)	1500

PPV = $a/(a + b)$ = (90/608) × 100 = 15%.

36. A 3

The number needed to treat (NNT) is calculated by 1/absolute benefit increase (ABI). The ABI is given by the difference in the outcomes between the two groups. This is 30% as quoted by the pharmaceutical representative, hence:

NNT = 1/30% = 100/30 = 3.3.

You therefore need to treat three patients with the new drug to prevent one annual hospitalisation. The NNT of the new drug also depends on the availability of other interventions and their NNTs, incremental cost and tolerability of the proposed intervention.

37. B Their abuse is strongly associated with personality disorders.

Magic mushrooms are small, and about 10–100 are typically used at a time. They are hallucinogenic and their active ingredients are psilocybin and psilocin. They have been used for magicoreligious reasons by the Indians of Mexico for many centuries. Almost half of misusers of magic mushroom have a personality disorder. Management of complications is symptomatic. They are not addictive and cannot be tested in the urine or hair.

38. C Headaches

Some adverse effects occur in up to 45% of patients early in the treatment programme. These include eye strain, blurred vision, eye irritation, and eye strain. Insomnia can occur particularly with late evening treatments. Rarely, manic mood swings and suicidal attempts have been noted as a result of treatment.

39. A Epilepsy can cause a decline in intellectual functioning.

Population-based studies reveal that learning disability is found in 30–40% of individuals with epilepsy, whereas the prevalence of epilepsy in the learning-disabled population is about 20–25%. It is higher in the more severely (IQ <50) than the mildly disabled (IQ 50–70), 30–50% and 15–20% respectively. It is unlikely that specific causal factors of epilepsy or cerebral palsy will ever be positively identified because these are non-specific clinical features of a brain disorder. Epileptic fits, if persistent, may produce brain damage and play a part in producing a progressive decline in the intellectual functioning of patients. Further apparent deterioration in intellectual functioning may be the result of excessively high anticonvulsant drugs.

40. D 9

The likelihood ratio of a positive test (LR+) is the ratio between the probability of a positive test in a person with the disease and the probability of a positive test in a person without the disease. It can also be expressed as:

LR+ = Sensitivity (1 − Specificity).

In the given example:

Sensitivity = 0.9/(1 − 0.9) = 0.9/0.1 = 9.

41. D 83%

To calculate post-test probability from likelihood ratios, it is necessary to determine the pre-test odds. The probability of a disease after a positive diagnostic test depends on the prevalence of the disease and the likelihood of a positive test result using the rating scale. The prevalence of anxiety in these patients, i.e. 20%, is taken as the pre-test probability.

Pre-test odds = Probability/(1 − Probability) = 20%/(1 − 20%) = 20/80 = 1/4.

Post-test odds = LR × Pre-test odds = 20 × 1/4 = 5.

Post-test probability = Odds/(1 + Odds) = 5/(1 + 5) = (5/6) × 100 = 83%.

42. C. 5

The NNT is the number of patients who take the new antidepressant drug for one additional patient to benefit, compared with the placebo in the given example. In this study, the response ratio is determined by a 50% drop in the MADRS scores from baseline. Of the 200 patients, 80, i.e. 40%, in the antidepressant group and 40, i.e. 20%, in the placebo group responded. This means that 20% (40% − 20%) additional patients in the antidepressant group responded compared with the placebo group. To translate this information into the NNT, we can use the formula:

NNT = 1/ABI (absolute benefit increase).

ABI = EER − CER (experimental event rate − control event rate).

EER - CER = 40% − 20% = 20%.

NNT = 1/20% = 5.

43. E Schizophrenia

Other contraindications include eating disorders and personality disorders.

44. D It may take different psychopathological forms.

Morbid jealousy (also known as Othello's syndrome) is a symptom rather than a diagnosis and therefore does not have a separate ICD-10 classification. It may lie anywhere on the spectrum from obsession or an overvalued idea to a delusion. A careful history and thorough mental state examination should help in finding out the nature and degree of the symptom, thus helping towards appropriate management. The most important association is alcohol misuse, although any substance misuse such as amphetamines should also be considered. Low self-esteem, schizophrenia and organic brain syndromes have also been associated with morbid jealousy. De Clerambault's syndrome is an erotomania in which the patient believes that an exalted person is in love with her or him.

# Answers: MCQs

45. B Assume non-normality and use non-parametric tests
If they haven't done so one should provide an explanation if they have checked for normality.

46. A The test has a high sensitivity.
This measures the percentage of people with the illness that the test correctly identifies. Specificity is the percentage of patients without the illness that the test identifies.

The PPV is the proportion of the patients whom the test identifies as having the illness that actually have it. NPV is the proportion of patients whom the test does not identify as having the illness that actually do not have it. Validity means that the test measures what it is supposed to.

47. A The odds ratio is also called the cross-product ratio.
This refers to the comparison of the odds of an event occurring in one group with that of it occurring in another group. It is a measure of the strength of an association calculated by comparing outcomes in exposed and non-exposed participants. An odds ratio of 1 is an equal chance of having or not having the disease. It is reported in case–control studies, but is not used to calculate the likelihood of developing a condition. If the condition is rare, the odds ratio equals the risk ratio.

48. B It is usually seen in bipolar II disorder.
Rapid cycling mood disorder occurs exclusively in bipolar disorder, usually in the bipolar II subtype. It is more common in females. Rapid cycling usually occurs at an early age and increases the risk of suicide attempts. Rapid cycling is defined as the occurrence of at least four episodes per year and it is not inherited.

49. E She can make an advance decision if she has a capacity to understand her illness, as well as the treatment process.
An 'advance decision' is a decision made by an individual, of all ages, who has a good mental capacity. It is the decision to refuse a particular treatment and is legally binding. The individual can revoke or change the advance decisions at a future date provided he or she possesses good mental capacity. It comes into force when the individual loses capacity to make a particular decision related to treatment.

A patient's wishes should be taken into consideration in administration of treatment, as far as possible. However, if the patient is detained under the Mental Health Act and the responsible clinician feels that a particular treatment is necessary for the protection of the patient and others, he can administer the appropriate treatment, unless it is ruled out by an advance decision..

50. C To combine the studies in a meta-analysis and produce a net effect
Multiple testing includes Bonferroni's correction or Tukey's post-hoc testing, effect size and Cohen's κ. Histograms can be used to study the normality of the data. The Mantel–Haenszel method provides a pooled odds ratio across the strata of fourfold tables. Meta-analysis is used to investigate the combination or interaction of a group of independent studies.

51. E Single blind

Blinding ensures that patients and doctors do not know which treatment is given. Single-blind studies reduce the potential biases of a patient's placebo response.

52. D A switch to mania was equal for antidepressants and placebo.

The US National Institutes for Mental Health (NIMH) sponsored STAR*D, which studied treatment alternatives to relieve depression and STEP-BD (Systematic Enhancement Programme for Bipolar Disorder) to look into the roles of antidepressants in acute bipolar depression. The patients included were already on a baseline mood stabiliser (i.e. lithium, divaloprex or carbamazepine), and there was an equal response rate of 25% in both groups (one received a placebo and other an antidepressant). About 10% switched to mania in both groups. The conclusion was that antidepressants were no better than placebo when added to a mood stabiliser for treating acute bipolar depression. The two antidepressants used in the STEP-BD trial were bupropion and paroxetine.

53. A An opportunity cost is defined as the cost of a decision in terms of the next best alternative; it occurs because human beings have endless needs and require resources to satisfy these needs.

Costs describe the total value of resources that are expended in the pursuance of the end. In the health-provision context, the direct cost of treatment programme X would include all identifiable equipment cost along with other costs such as project planning, building and premises, staff salaries, equipment administration, etc.

Indirect costs in the health-provision context would include patient-borne costs such as absence from work and other duties during the treatment period, loss of earnings and losses caused by treatment side effects, etc. The opportunity cost in the health provision context will include the value of other things, which are resources used by treatment programme X, that would have been spent in other ways such as other treatment programmes.

Intangible costs include discomfort, loss of independence, the allergic reaction to the medication and cosmetically unsightly scars.

54. C Patients with hospital addiction syndrome tend to become aggressive and may use sexual elements.

Hospital addiction syndrome is widely known as Munchausen's syndrome. In this condition, individuals become impostors as a defence against feelings of inferiority, and may masochistically play out a game with staff involving aggressive and sexual elements. This is perhaps to counter unconscious guilt and the psychological disintegration of the individual. A sick role was described by Parsons in 1951 derived from learning and role theories. Accident neurosis overlaps with post-traumatic stress but is not synonymous. Factitious disorder is characterised by physical or psychological symptoms that are feigned but not for gain. If it is for gain, it becomes malingering. In Munchausen's syndrome by proxy, physical (not psychological) symptoms are produced intentionally in others.

55. D It is the cumulative incidence

'Risk' (R) and 'prevalence' (P) in epidemiology do not have any units. The rapidity of disease occurrence is called the 'incidence rate'. Case/person time is the unit of the incidence rate (IR), which is also called the 'incidence density'. Risk is the proportion of unaffected individuals who may develop the disease over a specified period of time. It is also known as cumulative incidence.

R = New cases/Persons at risk

P = Cases/Population

IR = number of new cases in the population/person time (person-year is when a population is observed for 1 year for development of the disease).

56. E They include prospective designs.

In an RCT, participants are allocated to any branch of the trial by a process comparable to flipping a coin (i.e. heads goes to placebo and tails goes to intervention arm). The outcomes are clearly defined at the outset of the study and both arms are followed over a specified period of time to analyse the outcome. On average, the groups are identical except for the intervention, so any differences in analysis of outcome are attributable to the intervention. The RCT allows the rigorous evaluation of a single variable (i.e. drug vs placebo). It is always a prospective study design. It uses hypotheticodeductive reasoning (the null hypothesis) and potentially eliminates bias by comparing two almost identical groups, allowing for meta-analysis.

57. B Multiple regression using the least-square method

This is used to describe the numerical relationship of a dependent variable on several predictor variables. The term 'regression' means an equation that allows one variable called the target variable to be predicted from another variable, which is independent. Regression by the least-square method is used to analyse or describe a numerical relationship between two quantitative variables when the value of one variable can be predicted from the other (e.g. when determining the height from the age of the tree, age is the independent variable and height the dependent variable). Spearman's rank correlation coefficient, which is also known as the product–moment correlation coefficient, is used to assess the strength of the straight-line association between two continuous variables (price of petrol increasing as the distance from the town centre decreases, i.e. the nearer the petrol pump is to the town centre the more expensive the petrol).

58. C Two-sample (unpaired) Student's *t*-test (Mann-Whitney U-test)

This compares two independent samples drawn from the same population, e.g. to compare the height of boys with that of girls from a population sample. McNemar's test (paired) compares categorical data from two groups. The χ^2 test (unpaired data, also called 'independent' data) is used to compare more than two categorical data. One-sample (paired) Student's *t*-test (Wilcoxon's matched-pairs test) compares two sets of non-parametric observations from a single sample, e.g. comparing weights of infants before and after a meal.

59. E Two-way analysis of variance (by ranks)

This is used to test the influence or interaction of two different co-variables, in this case blood glucose and sex.

60. E Looking at various survival indices in one group over the study period

Kaplan–Meier survival analysis looks at one group. It is used to determine survival probabilities and proportions of participants surviving at the end of the study period, which helps to estimate cumulative survival probabilities. The Mantel–Haenszel test compares two unpaired (independent) groups. Cox's proportional hazard regression is used to compare three unmatched groups. Conditional proportional hazard regression is to compare two, three or more matched (paired) groups.

61. D Cost–utility analysis

This is used when we have different interventions with different outcomes and want to choose the best intervention in terms of the cost per quality-adjusted life-year (QALY) gained. It is the number of extra life-years obtained by an intervention and the value of the quality of life during those extra life-years. Resources in health services are limited. Economic analysis assesses the best available interventions and their benefits. Cost-minimisation analysis is used to find out the least costly intervention that achieves a similar magnitude of desired outcome. Cost-effective analysis is used to compare the cost of achieving a desired outcome within a limited budget. Cost–benefit analysis means benefits minus costs and is always considered in monetary terms. Sensitivity analysis is used to assess how robust the conclusion of any economic analysis is.

62. D Per-protocol analysis

The on-treatment analysis or the per-protocol analysis is an approach that uses only the data from patients who had complied sufficiently with the trial protocol. It creates bias because it excludes other participants from the analysis. The intention-to-treat analysis (which includes the drop-outs in one way or another in the final analysis) is therefore the best choice for analysis although per protocol could be done if necessary.

63. A Cronbach's α

This is used to measure internal consistency for tests with several parts or variables. Cronbach's α increases as the correlation between scale items increases. If it is >0.5, the correlation is moderate and, if >0.8, it is excellent.

κ, also known as chance-corrected proportional agreement statistics, measures interrater reliability. The intraclass correlation coefficient is used for the test measuring quantitative variables. It shows to what extent two continuous measures taken by different people, as well as two measures taken by same person on two different occasions, are related.

64. B Composite endpoint

The results of various studies are reported in terms of endpoints. A composite endpoint measures several endpoint outcomes using a prespecified algorithm. It is useful when a particular event occurs too frequently to be an endpoint and overcomes the problem of insufficient power in the study. The clinical endpoint measures direct clinical outcomes, e.g. mortality, survival. The surrogate endpoint measures a physical sign for a clinically meaningful endpoint. Surrogate markers are used in phases 1 and 2 of clinical trials. In an animal experimental set-up, humane endpoints are considered to reduce or terminate the pain and/or distress of the experimental animals by ending their life.

65. B Eliminating confounders

The null hypothesis suggests that there is no difference between two study groups. The aim of all studies is to be able to reject the null hypothesis in order to prove that an actual difference exists. Type 1 error (also called α) occurs when a false-positive result (i.e. there is a difference between the two groups) is obtained whereas in actuality there is no difference between the two groups. It usually occurs due to bias/confounders. A type 2 error (also called β) occurs when a null hypothesis is falsely rejected, i.e. although there is an actual difference in the two groups the study was unable to find one. This usually happens as a result of small sample size or if the measurement variance is too large. It can therefore be avoided by power calculation before the study.

66. D Type 2 error

In a meta-analysis, when the results of the underlying clinical trials are widely different, they are said to be heterogeneous. As the tests of heterogeneity used in a meta-analysis (Forest plot, χ2 statistics, z statistic, Galbraith's plot) have a limited statistical power, these tests are prone to type 2 error, i.e. they may falsely reject the presence of heterogeneity in the data in a meta-analysis.

67. D Two-sample Student's *t*-test

This is a hypothesis test to determine the mean when two random samples with independent observations have a normal distribution. The χ^2 test is used to find differences in proportions between two groups. McNemar's test is used to identify differences in proportions between two matched groups across two categories. The Mann–Whitney test is used to identify differences in medians between two independent groups. Wilcoxon's test is useful to identify differences in medians between two matched groups.

68. E Toxoplasmosis usually presents with focal neurological signs.

Viral, fungal and parasitic infections are common and bacterial invasions rare. They occur in about a third of the patients with HIV. The most common fungal infections are with cryptococci or *Candida albicans*. Aspergillosis or coccidioidomycosis is considered an uncommon infection. Ring-enhancing lesions on CT brain scans are diagnostic of *Toxoplasma gondii* infection. If detected early, there is a dramatic improvement in response to medication in *T. gondii* infection. Herpes zoster causes severe haemorrhagic encephalitis limited to the temporoparietal regions. Occasionally it also presents as an ascending myelitis.

69. B Double-blind study

In such a study design, both the participants and the investigators are blind to the treatments under investigation to avoid bias from them. The results from such studies are likely to be clinically relevant if they are statistically significant.

70. C 20%

After a first episode of schizophrenia, almost 20% live independently. Another 20% have no further episodes and 40% stay in employment and/or higher education; 50% will show some improvement.

71. B 1 month

The essential criteria for a diagnosis of ICD-10 non-organic insomnia include difficulty in either falling asleep or maintaining sleep. There is a constant preoccupation with lack of sleep and its consequences, causing marked distress. The sleep is non-restorative and of poor quality, which interferes with ordinary day-to-day activities. The aforementioned should happen at least three times a week for at least a month to fulfil the criteria of non-organic insomnia.

72. C Effect size

The effect size is the difference between two means divided by the standard deviation in controls. It is a measure of the strength of the relationship between two variables in a statistical population. The power is the ability to detect a difference between groups if still there. The larger the sample size, the more power a researcher has to detect the differences. The power is also defined as the probability of rejecting the null hypothesis when a true difference exists. The type 1 error is α and the type 2 error β.

73. C 2-fold

The presence of a personality disorder in a depressed patient can adversely affect the outcome of depression: it doubles the risk of poor outcome with any treatment for depression except electroconvulsive therapy (ECT).

74. D Monozygotic twins with OCD in the other sibling.

Obsessive–compulsive personality disorder (OCPD) is not a prominent risk factor for OCD, because the prevalence of OCPD in OCD and the general population is almost the same. In the adult group, men and women have equal prevalence, although adolescent boys have a higher prevalence. Single people are usually affected more often and this may indicate the difficulties in building relationships that people with OCD might experience. OCD is probably associated with abnormalities of serotonin (5-hydroxytryptamine or 5HT) as either a cause or an effect of these abnormalities. It may be associated with a possible genetic mutation in the human serotonin transporter gene (*hSERT*). The genetic factors account for 45–65% of OCD diagnoses in children.

75. E Schizotypal personality disorder

A poor prognosis in OCD is associated with coexisting schizotypal personality disorder. Others factors include yielding to compulsions, male gender, early age of onset, tics with OCD, hoarding, psychotic features, the need for hospitalisation, coexisting depression, delusional beliefs and the presence of overvalued ideas. Less avoidance gives a better prognosis. A good prognosis is indicated by good social and occupational adjustment.

76. B Fetal alcohol syndrome

Its clinical features include those described in the question.

77. A Catalepsy

This is characterised by perseveration of posture without any resistance to passive movements, and occurs in catatonia. This patient may have narcolepsy, which is characterised by irresistible excessive daytime sleepiness. It could be associated with cataplexy (falling as a result of sudden loss of muscle tone provoked by strong emotion), sleep paralysis (inability to move during the period between wakefulness and sleep) and hypnagogic hallucinations (between wakefulness and sleep). Sleep apnoea can also present as excessive daytime sleepiness.

78. D Huntington's disease

This is characterised by middle life onset with choreiform movements. The patient may become depressed early in the course of the illness, and withdrawn and isolated in the late stages. There may be personality changes and paranoid symptoms, but cognitive symptoms are usually late. It is inherited in an autosomal dominant fashion with complete penetrance. This patient does not fulfil the criteria of schizophrenia. Alzheimer's disease is unlikely to be present at this age with a movement disorder. Choreiform movements differentiate Huntington's disease from frontotemporal dementia, which is also rarely hereditary. Gilles de la Tourette's syndrome will not present with memory and paranoid symptoms.

79. C It is schizophrenia with learning disability.

'*Pfropf*' (German) means 'engrafted'. It is a kraepelinian concept: when schizophrenia presents admixed with learning disability. It is important to study the developing patterns and chronology of cognitive deficits and psychotic symptoms because they may point to the diverse underlying pathophysiology. This affects its overall management.

80. D Psychotic presentations are primarily of a hallucinatory rather than a delusional type.

Psychosis due to MS, such as an expansive delusional state (paranoid–hallucinatory), is common and neurological symptoms such as paraesthesia are sometimes incorporated as part of a paranoid delusional system. Depression is common and suicide is 14 times more common than in the general population. Intellectual deterioration occurs in around 50–66% of the patients. The onset of dementia is fairly sudden with confusion, memory loss and personality change. Verbal skills are relatively preserved till late in the disease process.

81. B The most common psychiatric presentation is depression with anergia.

The patients become depressed, listless, tired and dull, with marked lack of spontaneity and initiative. Depression responds well to removal of parathyroid adenomas, which are quite often the cause, although some patients need antidepressants. High levels of calcium can cause psychological disturbances. Psychosis occurs in around 5% of patients when it presents with acute delirium, hallucinations, paranoia and aggression. Diagnosis of hyperparathyroidism is usually delayed for several years because of its silent course.

82. E Temporal relationship

Other criteria include:

- Biological plausibility
- Coherence
- Experiment (reversibility)
- Analogy (consideration of alternative explanations)
- Specificity
- Strength of association.

83. B The effect of nicotine on dopamine release is similar to the effect of cocaine.

Dopamine release has an important role in so-called 'reward mechanisms' in our brain system. Nicotine's effect on dopamine release is similar to that of cocaine. Taking up of smoking in teenagers is more probably the result of psychosocial rather than biological reasons. In the UK, up to 25% of teenagers take up smoking by the age of 15. The prevalence of smoking is more frequent in single parents, divorced or separated individuals, drug users and prisoners. Higher rates are also seen in unemployed and homeless people. Smoking in women doubles the risk of ectopic pregnancy, along with increased risk of spontaneous abortions.

84. D Outburst of aggression and uncontrollable rage

'Pathological alcohol intoxication' is an extremely negative reaction to a small amount of alcohol that would not produce intoxication in most people. It is described as a sudden outburst of aggression, uncontrollable rage and often violent behaviour that is not typical of the person when sober. The legal definition of pathological intoxication is: it is a state in which a person's normal capacity to act or reason is impaired by alcohol or drugs. In ICD-10, the term 'pathological intoxication' applies only to alcohol. In some jurisdictions, pathological intoxication is a defence for specific-intent offences, whereas, in others, it is recognised as a defence for general-intent offences as well. Alcohol-induced amnesias ('blackouts') refer to transient states of amnesia after excessive drinking. Alcoholic hallucinosis includes hallucinations (mainly auditory) occurring in clear consciousness without autonomic hyperactivity when a person stops drinking after years of excessive drinking.

85. A A man's positive identity is contingent upon his relationships, care for others and altruistic behaviour.

A woman's self-esteem is more likely to be created and maintained by relationships, care of others and altruistic behaviour, whereas a male's self-esteem is more likely to be related to career achievement. A female's positive identity is thus more contingent on her relationships.

86. E There is at least a 7-day symptom-free phase after menstruation.

Of women with this disorder 20–40% consider it severe enough to seek medical help whereas for about 6% it is incapacitating during the premenstrual period. There is an increase in parasuicidal acts, suicides, accidents, violent crimes and shoplifting. The symptoms start mid-cycle, and increase in number and severity to maximum intensity up to the day before the onset of menstruation. This is followed by a rapid and complete resolution of symptoms. The symptoms are absent between menstruation and ovulation. Premenstrual syndrome (PMS) is also known as late luteal-phase dysphoric disorder. The syndrome does not improve with age and parity.

87. B Cornea of the eye

Kayser–Fleischer rings are dark rings that appear to encircle the iris of the eye. They are due to copper deposition in the cornea's Descemet's membrane in Wilson's disease. They do not occur in all people with Wilson's disease and may be visible only on slit-lamp examination.

88. A Frontal lobe

The frequency of neuropsychiatric symptoms is up to 90% in the frontal lobe, 50–55% in the temporal lobe, up to 60% in the pituitary, as much as 25% in the occipital lobes and up to 16% in parietal lobe dysfunction.

89. D It is characterised by hyposexuality.

Geschwind's syndrome is also known as the Gastaut–Geschwind syndrome; it is a personality syndrome. It is characterised by the behavioural phenomenon of circumstantiality in the form of excessive verbal output, stickiness and hypergraphia. There is altered sexuality, usually hyposexuality, and exaggerated cognitive and emotional responses. The presence of an unsettled, ongoing controversy over this syndrome has been acknowledged.

90. B Constipation-predominant group has higher anxiety and depression rates.

The constipation-predominant group demonstrates abnormal vagal cholinergic function indicated by R–R interval changes in deep breathing. The diarrhoea-predominant group has abnormal adrenergic function. Patients with one gastrointestinal symptom have lower rates of major depression than patients with two gastrointestinal symptoms. IBS is a common gastrointestinal condition that presents with episodes of stomach cramps, bloating, constipation and diarrhoea. The symptoms usually start between age 20 and 30 years. Most patients will have either constipation or diarrhoea or episodes of both. The exact cause of IBS is not known, but it is believed that there is an increased sensitivity of the entire gastrointestinal tract. The symptoms often occur during a stressful time or after eating certain types of food. IBS can be managed by making changes to diet and lifestyle, and taking antispasmodics such as hyoscine, mebeverine and peppermint oil.

91. A A graded increase in schizophrenia is seen with increasing maternal BMI.

A threefold increase in schizophrenia is seen in the highest maternal BMI category (>30). BMI is defined as the weight in kilograms divided by the square of the height in metres (kg/m2); a high BMI is associated with neural tube defects, and a normal BMI is 18.5–24.9. The predictors of obesity in adulthood include lower social class, a high maternal BMI before pregnancy, a high BMI during adolescence and early menarche.

92. A Episodic course of symptom severity

Group A β-haemolytic streptococci cause rheumatic fever, and an anti-neuronal antibody response to the bacteria is also directed at parts of the basal ganglia. The symptoms of OCD occur in 70% of cases of Sydenham's chorea. PANDAS was defined by five diagnostic criteria: abrupt onset, presence of OCD and/or tic disorder, prepubertal onset, episodic course of symptom severity, and dramatic exacerbations of symptoms temporarily associated with GABHS. An antigen labelled D8/17 on the surface of peripheral blood mononuclear cells has been shown to be a marker for the genetic tendency to generate abnormal antibodies to GABHS. The first-degree relatives of patients with PANDAS have higher rates of tic disorders and OCD.

93. A Conjugal paranoia

Pathological (delusional) jealousy is also known as Othello's syndrome, morbid jealousy, erotic jealousy, sexual jealousy, psychotic jealousy and conjugal paranoia. Folie-à-deux is an induced psychosis. Erotomania or De Clérambault's syndrome is a delusion of love. Ekbom's syndrome is delusional parasitosis.

94. C It is more common in women than in men.

L'illusion des sosies, also called Capgras' syndrome, is characterised by a delusion of doubles. Patients believe that the people known to them have been replaced by exact doubles. Facial processing in these patients is normal but the emotional concomitants of familiar face perception are disconnected from it. This leads to an anomalous affectless experience, which can be explained in the delusional beliefs. It usually occurs in the context of paranoid schizophrenia but also in other mental disorders. Nihilistic delusional disorder relates to Cotard's syndrome and is also called delire de negation. Folie-à-deux refers to the presence of an identical or similar mental disorder in two or more individuals who are usually members of a close family. Its treatment consists of separation, antipsychotics, individual and group psychotherapy, and family therapy. Severe self-neglect in elderly people is seen in Diogenes' syndrome.

95. D Onset of the disorder may occur any time before the age of 18.

Anxiety must last for a period of 4 weeks for a diagnosis to be made. In epidemiological studies, the disorder is more common in females; however, it is apparently equally common in clinic settings. Onset of the disorder may be as early as preschool and can occur any time before the age of 18. About 4% of children and young adolescents have the disorder. Typically there are periods of exacerbation and remission.

96. E Knife-blade atrophy

This is an extreme and global thinning of the gyri of the cerebral cortex, seen in the frontal and temporal lobes in Pick's disease. Frontotemporal dementias (including Pick's disease) are the second most common form of presenile dementias, and also comprise 7% of late life dementias. They have a broader and heterogeneous presentation. The behavioural symptoms are more prominent than cognitive decline. The affective symptoms include depression, apathy, emotional blunting and hypochondriasis. Pick's disease remains the archetypal frontotemporal dementia. The preliminary data indicate that the antidepressant trazodone, which blocks 5HT2-receptors may offer some benefit for behavioural disturbance.

97. A A strong desire or compulsion to use the substance

A strong desire or a compulsion to use the substance is included in ICD-10 not DSM-IV; the rest of the criteria are common to both classification systems.

98. B Intravenous diazepam

This is the preferred drug of choice. Chlordiazepoxide is ineffective in seizures. Anticonvulsant medications can be used if the cause of the seizures is difficult to establish in an emergency setting.

99. A Clinic privileges

Operant conditioning is reinforcement of a behaviour and, in this case, it is the drug-using behaviour that is reinforced by providing alternative incentives, depending on the user's abstinence from the target drug. These incentives can be monetary, vouchers, prizes or clinic privileges. The other options are not as effective as clinic privileges.

100. D 125 mg/L

If the patient is on valproate the dose should be increased to reach a peak level of 125 mg/L. Consider adding an antipsychotic if mania is severe. If the patient is already taking an anti-manic drug, check the levels and increase as appropriate to achieve serum lithium levels of 6.0–1.2 mmol/L. If the patient is on an antidepressant, it should be stopped.

101. D The pupils were bilaterally constricted and symmetrical.

Bilateral constricted pupils are a sign of opiate poisoning. The rest are features of Wernicke's encephalopathy. It consists of a classic triad of confusion, ataxia and ophthalmoplegia (especially of the lateral rectus muscles). The other clinical features include gaze palsies, short-term memory loss and confabulation. Wernicke's encephalopathy is caused by prolonged alcohol intake, which results in vitamin B_1 (thiamine) deficiency. This leads to lesions in the medial thalamic nuclei, mammillary bodies, superior cerebellar vermis, and the periaqueductal and periventricular brain-stem nuclei.

102. E Tic disorder

The following are also associated with OCD:

- Depression
- Simple phobias
- Social phobia
- Anxiety disorder
- Oppositional disorder
- ADHD
- Conduct disorder
- Separation anxiety disorder
- Enuresis and encopresis
- Eating disorders.

There is wide variety and range of co-morbidities in the adult population with OCD which are comparable with adults who had a childhood onset of OCD. Tics are found in almost 30% and anxiety disorders in 26–75 %, and depressive disorder in 25–62% of children with OCD.

103. D 11–14 years

Seizures affect about a quarter of autistic individuals with generalised learning disability and about 5% of autistic individuals with a normal IQ. Seizures often begin in adolescence. The peak age for onset of seizures is 11–14 years. By contrast, when individuals with a generalised learning disability but with no autistic problems develop seizures, the onset is usually in early childhood rather than adolescence.

104. E The disorder may continue into adulthood.

For a diagnosis, the child should have eaten non-nutritive substances for more than 1 month. There is no aversion to food. It is more commonly seen in younger children. It rarely continues into adulthood, but it is possible. Vitamin and mineral deficiencies are not common and it is brought to attention because of general medical complications.

105. D Median age of onset for motor tics is 6–7 years.

This condition presents with multiple motor and one or more vocal tics. Onset of the disorder in all patients is below the age of 18 and may be as early as 2 years. Coprolalia (complex vocal tics involving uttering of obscenities) is present in less than 10% of cases of Gilles de la Tourette's syndrome. It affects boys twice as much as girls according to community studies.

106. B Children's Depression Inventory (CDI) has self, parent and teacher report forms.

The only self-reported scale accepted and validated for children and adolescents is the MFQ with 37 items. The scales mainly used in adolescents are the CES-D and BDI.

107. B Almost three-quarters of children are found to be securely attached.

The strange situation experiment was devised by Ainsworth and Wittig in 1969. Three types were observed during the experiment (**Table 3.6**).

Table 3.6 Classification of attachments

Category	Description	%
Type A: anxious–avoidant	Baby largely ignores mother because of indifference towards her. No or few signs of distress when mother leaves. Ignores her when she arrives. Comforted as easily by a stranger as by the mother	15
Type B: securely attached	Baby plays happily when mother is present. Distressed when mother leaves and play is reduced. Stranger can provide only limited comfort	70
Type C: anxious–resistant	Baby cries more, and becomes very distressed when mother leaves. Seeks comfort when mother returns but also shows anger and resists contact. Resists strangers' contact, i.e. treats mother and stranger differently	15

A type D category has also been identified: insecure–disorganised in which the baby lacks goals, shows contradictory behaviour and even shows fear of the mother. Type D has been linked to infant maltreatment, hostile caregiving, maternal loss through separation/divorce/death and maternal depression.

108. E Parents with other mental health problems

NICE recommends that services should use methods to identify children at risk of developing conduct problems. Vulnerable parents should be identified, where appropriate antenatally. There are various risk factors which mainly include parents having a history of residential care, drug or alcohol problems, or any mental illness, having ongoing or history of contact with the criminal justice system or mothers younger than 18 years who were themselves maltreated in their childhood.

109. C Moderate learning disability

Learning disability is a condition of arrested or incomplete development of the mind resulting in impairment of intelligence, i.e. cognitive, language, motor and social abilities. It is classified into IQ categories as follows: mild 50–69, moderate 35–49, severe 20–34 and profound <20 (based on ICD-10).

110. B Around 1% of adolescents aged >15 years have the disorder.

Enuresis is repeated voiding of urine, which can happen during the night or daytime into the bed or clothes. It can also be intentional. For a diagnosis, the chronological or mental age of the child must be ≥5 years. Around 1% of adolescents aged >15 years have the disorder. It affects 5–10% of 5 year olds and 3–5% of 10 year olds. Approximately 75% of children with the disorder have a first-degree biological relative who has had the disorder.

111. C Vineland's Social Adaptive Behaviour Test

Disability shows how much a person could not adapt to his or her social environment. This is assessed by using social maturity or adaptation scales. One such scale is Vineland's Social

Maturity Scale or Vineland's Social Adaptive Behaviour Test. Other tests mentioned here are neuropsychological tests as well as intelligence tests.

112. E Phenylketonuria

This is the most common inborn error of amino acid metabolism due to deficiency of phenylalanine hydroxylase. It leads to increased phenylalanine levels in the body. Guthrie's test is useful in detecting phenylketonuria (PKU). which is an autosomal recessive disorder caused by mutation in the gene that is responsible for the synthesis of phenylalanine hydroxylase. This can lead to microcephaly, severe learning disability and epilepsy. Early identification helps to restrict diet with phenylalanine so intellectual disability is drastically reduced. The neonatal screening programmes use Guthrie's test to detect PKU in newborns.

113. E Onset at young age

Good prognostic factors are late onset, obvious precipitating factors, acute onset, good pre-morbid personality, mood symptoms, being married, family history of mood disorder, good support system and positive symptoms. Poor prognostic factors are young onset, absence of precipitating factors, insidious onset, poor pre-morbid personality, withdrawn and autistic behaviour, being single/divorced/widowed, family history of schizophrenia, negative symptoms, many relapses and no remission in 3 years.

114. B Self-injurious behaviour is more common in mild than moderate learning disability.

Aggressive behaviour is a common problem among learning-disabled individuals. Aggression is often a feature of the psychosis; depression or antisocial personality disorder is observed in genetic disorders such as the fragile X, Prader–Willi and Klinefelter's syndromes. Learned aggression through the imitation of aggressive models or as a function of communication is also found relatively frequently among people with learning disability. Self-injurious behaviour occurs more often among people with severe learning disability (IQ <50). It occurs most frequently between the age of 10 and 30 years, with a peak between 15 and 20 years. It is related to genetic and organic disturbances and also adverse environmental and developmental conditions. Some psychiatric disorders such as depression may also elicit self-injurious behaviour.

115. E Social anxiety, shyness, gaze aversion, autism, inattention, hyperactivity, depression

Fragile X syndrome presents with shyness, gaze aversion and marked anxiety in social situations. Autism, depression, inattention and hyperactivity might be present. Williams' syndrome presents with social disinhibition with indiscriminate relating. Inattention, hyperactivity, fear, phobias and anxiety may be evident. In the Prader–Willi syndrome, there is excessive eating (hyperphagia), lability, under-activity and self-injury (skin picking). There may also be non-food obsessions and compulsions. Cri-du-chat is characterised by an infantile, high-pitched, cat-like cry. There may be stereotypies, repetitive movements and self-injury behaviour. Inattention and hyperactivity might be present. Individuals with Down's syndrome present as stubborn with non-compliant behaviour, together with being argumentative, overactive and inattentive. In the Smith–Magenis syndrome, there is self-injurious behaviour, aggression, hyperactivity, self-hugging and sleep disturbances with stereotypies (usually with the mouth).

116. C Mathematics disorder

Various DSM-IV learning and skills disorders in childhood include: reading disorder, mathematics disorder, disorders of written expression, developmental coordination disorder, expressive language disorder, mixed receptive–expressive language disorder, phonological disorder and stuttering.

117. C Stockholm syndrome

This is a term coined by the criminologist Nils Bejerot. It was introduced to describe the unexpected reactions of hostages both during and after an armed raid on the Sveriges Kredit Bank in Stockholm in 1973. Over a 6-day period, it was noted that the four hostages (including three women) began to develop positive feelings towards their male captors and vice versa. After their release, the hostages even set up a fund to pay for their captors' legal defence fees. The other options are all possible effects of being taken hostage. Patty Hearst refers to a similar reaction whereby, despite being taken hostage by a liberation group, the victim (Patty Hearst) agreed to be a member and join them in their cause. However, she displayed no subsequent sympathy for their cause and did not seek to defend their actions. She stated that she chose consciously to stay with her captors to ensure her survival.

118. D 70%

The clinical features of autism include delay in spoken language. For children with the full autistic syndrome, approximately 70% eventually acquire useful speech. Children who have not done so by age 5 are unlikely to do so subsequently. About 10% of autistic individuals go through a phase in adolescence when they lose language skills. This decline is not progressive but the lost skills are not generally regained.

119. B An adverse environment shared by captors and captives

The following are pre-conditions for the development of Stockholm syndrome:

- An extended and emotionally charged event
- An adverse environment shared by captors and captives (e.g. lack of warmth, food, shelter)
- Opportunities for a bond to develop (to counter this guards may be frequently moved to different hostages)
- When threats to life are not fulfilled (e.g. 'mock' executions)
- When the hostages, deprived of their usual support, have a high level of dependence on the hostage takers even for the most basic needs
- When the hostages are perceived by their captors as personalised human beings (to avoid this, in some incidents, hostages are 'dehumanised' by being given pseudonyms or numbers and treated as animals or 'aliens').

120. A It can be used in an actuarial manner.

The HCR-20 is a structured professional judgement tool, although there are item scores that can be totalled. Most research studies of the HCR-20 use the scores in an actuarial manner by adding the score items. The real strength of the HCR-20 lies in its use to guide clinical judgement about risk and therefore about risk management. No tool can accurately predict violence risk. However, the HCR-20 is a good predictor of violent and non-violent offences by male psychiatric patients released from medium secure units. The HCR-20 combines static (historical) and dynamic (clinical) items. Evidence suggests that it has consistent international reliability and validity. It consists of:

- Ten historical factors: previous violence, young age at first violence, relationship instability, employment problems, substance use problems, major mental illness, psychopathy, early maladjustment, personality disorder and prior supervision failure
- Five clinical factors: lack of insight, negative attitudes, active symptoms, impulsivity and

unresponsiveness to treatment
- Five risk management items: management plans lack feasibility, exposure to destabilisers, non-compliance, stress and lack of personal support.

121. C It is based on cognitive–behavioural theory.

The work of Finklehor and Araji has been particularly influential in the development of cognitive–behavioural treatment for sex offenders in both the USA and the UK. This four-stage model offers the theory that sex offenders will commit sexual offences only when they have moved through all of the following four stages:

1. Motivation to abuse sexually
2. Overcoming internal inhibitions, e.g. developing cognitive distortions or misusing substances
3. Overcoming external inhibitions, e.g. a paedophile may offer to baby sit
4. Overcoming the resistance of the victim, e.g. offering bribes or threatening violence.

SOTP therapy is usually facilitated using group therapy, but individual sessions are carried out occasionally. It is not medication based, but some participants may be on anti-libidinal treatments combined with group therapy. SOTP therapy can be carried out in the community (usually by probation), in prisons and more frequently within secure mental health units, which are more geared to dealing with sex offenders with mental health difficulties.

122. D Multidimensional family therapy should consist of 12–15 weekly sessions.

Drug and alcohol abuse in children and young people is thought to be a complex phenomenon with intertwined personal issues, interpersonal relationships and family environment.

Multidimensional family therapy (MDFT) usually involves 12–15 structured sessions over a period of 12 weeks. It looks at a child's education and social behaviour, the parents' parenting skills and the interactions of the parents and child. The theory is that a youth's problematic behaviour is thought to serve some function within the family dynamics. The behavioural pattern adapted by family members to satisfy their relational needs may, in turn, maintain the young person's behavioural problems; it is the basis of family functional therapy (FFT). On average, there are 8–12 1-hour sessions, usually given over 3-month period.

Brief strategic family therapy (BSFT) is based on the theory that family members are interdependent; patterns of family interactions affect behaviour of individual family members and BSFT addresses these patterns of interaction to change the behaviour of the adolescents. The average duration is 12–16 sessions given over a 3- to 4-month period.

123. B High rates of psychotic disorder exist in prisoners remanded for psychiatric reports.

Psychiatric symptoms are common in the first 2 months of imprisonment. Between a third and a half have ICD-10-classifiable psychiatric disorders. Personality disorder and substance abuse are the most common psychiatric diagnoses. In sentenced prisoners, the prevalence of a psychotic disorder is similar to that in the general population.

124. E Pre-existing heart disease

Disulfiram inhibits aldehyde dehydrogenase and leads to accumulation of acetaldehyde after drinking alcohol. This can lead to extremely unpleasant physical effects such as facial flushing, headache, tachycardia, nausea and vomiting, arrhythmias and hypotension. Disulfiram is contraindicated in patients with coronary artery disease, cardiac failure, hypertension, and a history of cerebrovascular disease, psychosis, severe personality disorder and suicide risk.

125. A Amphetamine, if snorted

However, it will be classed as a class A drug if it is prepared for injection.

Table 3.7 Classification of illicit drugs	
Class	Drugs
Class A	Ecstasy, LSD, heroin, cocaine, crack cocaine, magic mushrooms, amphetamine (if prepared for injection)
Class B	Amphetamines, cannabis, methylphenidate, pholcodine
Class C	Tranquillisers, some painkillers, γ-hydroxybutyrate, ketamine

126. E Young people in possession will receive a reprimand, final warning or charge if caught for the first time.

An adult in possession will be arrested, fined or served a penalty. Cannabis was reclassified from class C to class B in 2009. The maximum penalty for possession of cannabis is 2 years' imprisonment and, for supplying, producing and trafficking, 14 years. A young person in possession will receive a reprimand, final warning or charge if caught for the first time.

127. A It is classified as a hypochondriacal disorder in the ICD-10.

Dysmorphophobia (body dysmorphic disorder) is classified as a form of hypochondriasis. It has been defined as 'a subjective feeling of ugliness or physical defect which the patient feels is noticeable to others, although his or her appearance is within normal limits'. The disorder consists of distressing and/or impairing preoccupation with a non-existent or slight defect in appearance. Dysmorphophobia can be delusional in nature, but more frequently presents as an overvalued idea. In a study of patients presenting to a plastic surgeon for cosmetic rhinoplasty the following findings were evident:

- As a group they were more disfigured than a control group.
- Forty per cent showed a disorder of personality.
- There was no relationship between the degree of deformity and the amount of psychological disturbance.

Body dysmorphic disorder occurs more frequently in late adolescence. Three-quarters of patients are women and most are either single or divorced.

128. B Hyperschemazia

This is the perceived magnification of body parts. It can occur with a variety of organic and mental disorders. When a part of the body is painful, it may feel larger than normal. When there is partial paralysis of a limb, the affected segment feels heavy and large. This is seen in Brown–Séquard paralysis when the side with extrapyramidal signs demonstrates hyperschemazia. It also occurs in non-organic disorders, e.g. hypochondriasis, depersonalisation and conversion disorder. Another example is the disturbance of body image in anorexic patients when they believe that they are fat in spite of severe weight loss. Aschemazia or hyposchemazia refers to the perception of body parts as absent or diminished, respectively. Paraschemazia refers to a feeling that parts of the body are distorted, twisted or separated from the rest of the body. It can occur in epileptic aura and migraine, and with hallucinogenic use. Asyndesis refers to a lack of adequate connections between successive thoughts. Kinaesthetic hallucination is a type of tactile hallucination. It refers to muscles and joints such that the patient feels that his or her limbs are pulled, moved or twisted. Metamorphosis is synonymous with dysmegalopsia, and refers to the description of objects that are irregular in shape. Dysmegalopsia is further divided into micropsia (objects smaller than their actual size), macropsia or megalopsia (objects larger than their actual size), and porropsia (retreat of objects into the distance without any change in size). Phantom limb refers to the condition when the patient feels the sensation that an amputated or missing limb is still part of his or her body, moving appropriately with other parts of his or her body. It is considered the most common organic somatic hallucination. Phantom sensations also occur after removal of other body parts.

129. B Dialectical behaviour therapy

This was developed to treat women with borderline personality disorder who were chronically parasuicidal. The approach is based on Linehan's biosocial theory that borderline personality disorder is caused by pervasive emotional dysregulation. Self-harm is considered to be a maladaptive solution to overwhelming, intensely painful emotions. Dialectical behaviour therapy (DBT) is the only empirically supported treatment for adults with multiple mental health problems presenting a risk of suicide. In a 2-year randomised controlled trial, DBT reduced suicidal behaviour, inpatient days and anger ratings compared with the usual treatment.

130. B One in which associations can be established but not the causation

Experimental studies include meta-analysis, systematic reviews, randomised controlled trials (RCTs), economic analysis of RCTs, uncontrolled trials, cluster trials, cross-over trials and n-of-1 trials. The observational studies are cohort studies, case–control studies, clinical audit, qualitative studies and surveys. RCTs are considered the gold standard in medical research.

Answers: EMIs

131. H Lewy body dementia

REM sleep behaviour disorder can appear years before the onset of Lewy body dementia and parkinsonism. It is the second most common form of dementia and shares many features with Alzheimer's disease. It starts at an early age, fluctuates in severity and progresses more rapidly. It is associated with parkinsonian features, sensitivity to antiemetics and antipsychotics, and visual hallucinations. There are Lewy bodies (intracytoplasmic inclusion bodies, α-synuclein) in the cerebral cortex, although they are also present in the subcortical region (as in Parkinson's disease) and can include neuritic plaques (as in Alzheimer's disease). There is a reduced cerebral metabolic rate for glucose in the posterior cingulate, parietal, prefrontal area similar to Alzheimer's dementia.

132. F Hypoactive delirium

Slow speech, lethargy, decreased alertness, sluggishness, decreased motor activity, staring and apathy are characteristic of hypoactive delirium. It is usually associated with metabolic disturbance, and is usually seen in hypercapnia (high levels of CO_2 in the blood) and hepatic encephalopathy. A reduced level of consciousness, intellectual impairment and personality changes characterise hepatic encephalopathy.

133. D Extradural haemorrhage

Head injuries causing skull fracture and leading to laceration of the middle meningeal artery and the accompanying dural sinuses are the most common aetiology. In extradural haemorrhage (EDH), 20–50% of patients have the classic lucid interval when a patient doesn't have any symptoms and is almost normal. The force resulting in the head injury might result in altered consciousness. After recovering consciousness (lucid interval), the EDH expands further and produces the mass effect of the haemorrhage, resulting in increased intracranial pressure, decreasing level of consciousness and later herniation syndrome.

134. A Cortical dementia

The symptomatology in dementia depends on the site of brain affected, i.e. cortical or subcortical. Most dementias are cortical, characterised by plaques and tangles (hallmark of Alzheimer's disease) in the cortices. Initial symptoms in cortical dementias include difficulties with one's memory, reasoning, problem-solving skills and language. Alzheimer's disease and FTD (frontotemporal dementia), which are 'cortical dementias', mainly present with amnesia, apraxia, agnosia and aphasia (4As).

135. G Late-onset schizophrenia

The symptom profile of late-onset schizophrenia is similar to that of earlier-onset schizophrenia. Formal thought disorder and negative symptoms are uncommon in patients with onset of psychosis after age 60. Almost half of these patients have mixed depressive–anxiety symptoms with confusion, catatonia and agitation. Compared with early onset schizophrenia, the late-onset form has less affective flattening and formal thought disorder, and a better prognosis. There is a higher incidence of visual, tactile and olfactory hallucinations, delusions of partition, persecution and auditory hallucinations, which can be a running commentary by a third person and accusatory.

Answers: EMIs

136. F Multiple linear regression

This is used for predicting the dependent variable from two or more independent variables. It attempts to model the relationship between two or more explanatory variables and a response variable by fitting a linear equation to observed data.

137. G Pearson's correlational coefficient

This is also known as Pearson's product–moment correlation coefficient. It is a correlational coefficient for two normally distributed variables. It shows linear correlation between two variables and gives a value between +1 and −1 inclusive.

138. H Proportional Cox's regression

This is also referred to as proportional hazard regression analysis and is used to assess survival or other time-related events. It is a type of logistic regression in which independent variables are related to the logarithm of the incidence rate of outcome by including a time factor.

139. I Simple linear regression

This is useful when there are two variables, one independent (X) and one dependent (Y), i.e. change in X causes a change in Y.

140. J Spearman's rank correlation coefficient

This is also known as Spearman's ρ and Pearson's correlation coefficient between ranked variables. It is a correlational coefficient in which one variable is normally distributed and the other is categorical or non-normally distributed. It assesses how well the relationship between two variables can be explained using a monotonic function. It is appropriate for continuous and discrete variables including ordinal variables.

141. D Nominal data

This means three or more unique categories bearing no mathematical relationship to each other.

142. C Gaussian distribution

A normal or gaussian distribution is characterised by the bell-shaped curve. The data in this distribution can be described by the mean and standard deviation. It is a continuous distribution function that approximates the exact binomial distribution of events.

143. F Ordinal data

This means that there is an order inherent in the measurement scale but it is not simply quantifiable. The categories for ordinal data have a natural order.

144. E 46%

The pooled analysis strongly suggests that there are susceptible loci on chromosomes 6p, 8p, 13q and 229. The last two may also be associated with bipolar affective disorder. The average lifetime risk is 5–10% among first-degree relatives of patients with schizophrenia. The risk increases to 46% when both parents have schizophrenia.

145. F 55%

Studies have consistently shown that women with a previous history of postpartum psychosis or bipolar disorder have a 20–30% risk of puerperal recurrence. This risk rises to >50% when family history is also a contributory factor.

146. B 8%

A family history of schizophrenia is a strong risk factor for this condition. This risk correlates with the closeness of the relationship. The risk of developing schizophrenia with a positive family history is given in **Table 3.8**.

Table 3.8 Prevalence of schizophrenia with a positive family history

Population	Prevalence (%)
General population	1
Non-twin sibling of a schizophrenic patient	8
Child with one parent having schizophrenia	12
Dizygotic twin of a patient with schizophrenia	12
Child with both parents having schizophrenia	40
Monozygotic twin of a patient with schizophrenia	47

147. B Ataque de nervios

This is a dissociative trance disorder that usually follows an acutely stressful event, e.g. a death. It is usually brief in duration with a trance-like state characterised by narrowing of awareness, peripheral distortions, depersonalisation, loss of consciousness, partial or global amnesia, anxiety, somatic complaints and depression.

148. D Brain fog

This is also known as brain fog syndrome and resembles anxiety, depression or somatoform disorders. The patient complains of reduced concentration, poor memory, blurred vision, headache, neck pain, and feeling pressure, heat or burning.

149. F Koro

This is also called 'genital retraction syndrome'. Prodromal depersonalisation usually occurs and the person takes elaborate measures to prevent the penis retracting. The female equivalent is fear or delusion that the labia or nipples are retracting, but this occurs rarely. There is no specific association with other mental disorders. However, phobic anxiety disorders, depression, schizophrenia and depersonalisation syndromes are described. It has been described in Malaysia, the Middle East, China, India, Singapore and Israel.

Some other culture-bound syndromes are shown in **Table 3.9**.

Table 3.9 Culture-bound syndromes

Syndrome	Culture	Main features
Koro	South and east Asia	Sudden and intense anxiety that the penis (or the vulva and nipples in women) will recede into the body, possibly causing death
Brain fag	West Africa	Experienced by students in response to the stress of schooling. Difficulty in memory, thinking, concentration, fatigue of the brain and somatic symptoms
Amok	Malaysia	A dissociative episode characterised by a period of brooding, followed by an outburst of violent, aggressive or homicidal behaviour
Ataque de nervios	Latinos from Caribbean	An idiom of distress includes uncontrollable shouting, attacks of crying, trembling, heat in the chest rising into the head, aggression and a sense of being out of control. It often follows a stressful event related to the family

150. H Non-competitive inhibition of acetylcholinesterase

Donepezil is an acetylcholinesterase (AChE) inhibitor causing the inhibition of the enzyme acetylcholinesterase. It is a reversible, non-competitive, acetylcholinesterase inhibitor, and leads to an increase in acetylcholine and thus a heightened cholinergic action.

151. D Competitive inhibition of acetylcholinesterase, E Nicotinic receptor modulation

Galantamine acts on both AChE and nicotinic acetylcholine receptors (nAChRs). The reduced nAChR's expression and activity is known to contribute towards the reduction of the central cholinergic neurotransmission in Alzheimer's disease. Galantamine acts as a competitive, reversible inhibitor of AChE and causes an allosteric regulation of nAChRs.

152. F NMDA antagonist

Memantine belongs to a class of drugs called NMDA-receptor antagonists. NMDA receptors are a subtype of glutamate receptors. Glutamate is an excitatory neurotransmitter which can be neurotoxic. By non-competitively blocking NMDA receptors, memantine can reduce glutamate-induced neurotoxicity.

153. F Flooding, G Self-harm

Some symptoms in depressed elderly patients are more striking compared with younger people, e.g. severe retardation, agitation, nihilistic delusions, delusions of poverty and physical illness. Depression itself is sometimes not conspicuous and may be masked by physical symptoms.

154. B Emotional abuse, C Falls, D Financial abuse

Abuse and neglect of elderly people by their family or other carers are issues of increasing concern to healthcare staff and statutory bodies. High-risk factors include dementia, the carer and abused

155. C Falls

Vascular dementia is the second most common type of dementia. It is slightly more common in men than in women. Its onset is usually in the seventh or eighth decade. It is often acute and follows a stroke. Transient ischaemic attacks (TIAs) and mild strokes may occur frequently.

156. B Amphetamines

They cause elated mood, over-talkativeness, overactivity, insomnia, dryness of lips, mouth and nose, and anorexia. Prolonged use of high doses of amphetamines may result in repetitive stereotyped behaviour and paranoid psychosis.

157. E Heroin

Opioids such as heroin, morphine and codeine, and synthetic analgesics such as pethidine, methadone and dipipanone, interact with opioid receptors. Heroin has a powerful euphoric effect when taken intravenously. In addition to analgesia, opioids produce respiratory depression, constipation, reduced appetite and low libido.

158. C Cannabis

Its clinical effects vary with the dose, the person's expectations and mood, and the social setting. It tends to give a 'high' and exaggerate the pre-existing mood of exhilaration or depression. Its adverse effects include irritation of the respiratory tract, anxiety, paranoid ideation, and toxic confusional states and psychosis.

159. H Selective mutism

This was formerly known as elective mutism. It is the persistent failure to speak in specific social situations despite speaking appropriately in other settings. The symptoms must last for at least 1 month for a diagnosis to be made. It usually starts before the age of 5 years and is rare (<1%) in the community. It is more common in girls.

160. A Attention deficit hyperactivity disorder (ADHD)

There are three subtypes of ADHD: inattentive, hyperactive/impulsive and combined. The most common overlap of symptoms of ADHD is with conduct disorder and oppositional defiant disorder. Stimulants are not contraindicated if co-morbid Gilles de la Tourette's syndrome is present; however, caution is advised. Medication is more effective than behavioural strategies. The point prevalence of ADHD is about 5%.

161. F Enuresis in 5-year-old children

Enuresis is repeated voiding of urine, which can happen during the night- or daytime into the bed or clothes. It can also be intentional. For a diagnosis, the chronological or mental age of the child must be ≥ 5 years. Around 1% of adolescents aged >15 years have the disorder. It affects 5–10% of 5 year olds and 3–5% of 10 year olds.

Table 3.10 gives a rough estimate of the prevalence of disorders.

Table 3.10 Prevalence of childhood disorders

Disorder	Prevalence[a] (%)
Anxiety disorders	8–12
Depression in adolescents	3–8
Bipolar	1
Depression in prepubertal children	1–2
Developmental coordination disorder	6
Dysthymia	2
Encopresis in 5-year-olds	1
Major depression in children	2
Major depression in adolescents	2–5
Obsessive–compulsive disorder (adolescents)	2
Separation anxiety disorder	4
Social phobias	2–4
Gilles de la Tourette's syndrome	3

[a]Prevalence rates may vary in different studies.

162. F Risk of Sexual Violence Protocol (RSVP)

This is a structured professional judgement tool, which has a similar format to the HCR-20. It allows the user to formulate the risk of sexual violence, using a number of appropriate risk factors. The RSVP has essentially replaced the SVR-20 (Sexual Violence Risk-20). It puts more emphasis on psychological risk factors and the development of case management plans. It is therefore considered to be more suited for evaluations conducted by sex offender specialists or for treatment purposes.

163. A Historical, Clinical, Risk Management 20 (HCR-20), E Psychopathy Check List – Revised (PCL-R)

The concept of psychopathy is referred to by Hare's Psychopathy Checklist (actuarial tool). The cluster of traits that Hare describes as a syndrome of psychopathy includes those that will lead to increased risk of harm. Some of the traits mentioned include: lack of empathy, dominance, forcefulness, lack of anxiety, lack of guilt, impulsivity, sensation seeking, superficial charm, pathological lying and manipulation.

Psychopathy as described by the PCL-R is strongly correlated with the risk of future violence. The PCL-R has a total score of 40. In the USA, a score of 30 is the cut-off for diagnosis of psychopathy; in the UK this cut-off is ≥25.

The HCR-20 would be the most appropriate violence risk assessment tool (structured professional judgement) to formulate risk of violence. The presence of psychopathy is one of the historical factors in the HCR-20.

164. D Millon Clinical Multi-axial Inventory (MCMI)

This is a self-report questionnaire to assess personality disorder. It is never used in isolation to diagnose someone with a personality disorder, but may offer a foundation for carrying out further assessments. Other self-report questionnaires for personality assessment include the Personality Disorder Questionnaire (PDQ-IV) and the Wisconsin Personality Inventory (WISPI).

165. I Violence Risk Appraisal Guide (VRAG)

This is specifically aimed at predicting violent reoffending in a community setting. It would be appropriate to consider the SARA; however, this is not an actuarial tool, but a structured one.

The VRAG is an actuarial tool that involves reading records, leading to assignment of a score to 12 items, which are processed to yield a percentage risk of reoffending. It contains the following historical items:

- PCL-R
- Elementary school difficulties
- Personality disorder
- Younger age
- Separated from parents before age 16
- Never married
- Absence of schizophrenia (presence decreases risk)
- Victim injury
- Alcohol abuse
- Female victim
- Failed conditional release/supervision order
- History of non-violent offence.

166. C Matrix 2000, G Sexual Offending Risk Appraisal Guide (SORAG)

These are both actuarial tools to assess sexual offending. The SORAG is a 14-item tool that incorporates the PCL-R. The Matrix 2000 assesses the statistical likelihood of reoffending by just convicted sex offenders who are adult males. The Matrix 2000 is used mainly by the national probation service and the police.

167. A Angelman's syndrome

Table 3.11 Chromosomal abnormalities and the resulting syndromes

Chromosomal abnormality	Syndrome	Birth rate (/1000)
15q12 deletion, maternally inherited	Angelman's syndrome	0.033–0.066
15q12 deletion, paternally inherited	Prader–Willi syndrome	0.07
4p deletion	Wolf–Hirschorn syndrome	Rare; two-thirds female
5p deletion	Cri-du-chat syndrome	0.02 70% female but more males survive

168. G Smith–Magenis syndrome

Table 3.12 Chromosomal abnormalities and the resulting syndromes

Chromosomal abnormality	Syndrome	Birth rate (/1000)
16p deletion, autosomal dominant	Rubenstein–Taybi syndrome	0.008
17q deletion	Smith–Magenis syndrome	0.04

169. D Edwards' syndrome

Table 3.13 Chromosomal abnormalities and the resulting syndromes

Chromosomal abnormality	Syndrome	Birth rate (/1000)
Trisomy 13	Patau's syndrome	0.2
Trisomy 18	Edwards' syndrome	0.3 M:F = 3:1
Trisomy 21: 94% non-disjunction 3–5% translocation 1–3% mosaic	Down's syndrome	1.4 Varies with maternal age from 1/1400 at 25 to 1/46 for age ≥45

170. C DiGeorge's (velocardiofacial) syndrome

Table 3.14 Chromosomal abnormalities and resulting syndromes

Chromosomal abnormality	Syndrome	Birth rate (/1000)
Chromosome 21 X-linked, mostly female	Aicardi's syndrome	
22q11.2	DiGeorge's (velocardiofacial) syndrome	0.16–0.25
Xq27	Fragile X syndrome	1 (male birth)
45,XO (60%) XX/XO (15%) Isochromosome Xq or Xp (10%) Xdel or Xring or Y abN (15%)	Turner's syndrome	1 (female)
47,XXY	Klinefelter's syndrome	1/500 (men)

171. I Williams' syndrome

Table 3.15 Chromosomal abnormalities and resulting syndromes

Chromosomal abnormality	Syndrome	Birth rate (/1000)
3q26.3	Cornelia de Lange's syndrome (Amsterdam dwarfism)	
7q11.2 autosomal dominant	Williams' syndrome	0.13
Autosomal dominant, incomplete penetrance (50%), sporadic mutation in the fibroblast growth factor gene	Apert's syndrome	0.00625
Autosomal recessive, almost 50% chromosome 11q13 gene (mostly whites), <20% 16q21 and 15q22, 3p13 possibly implicated	Laurence–Moon–Biedl syndrome	0.008

172. B Play the winner

In this approach, the first participant is allocated by simple randomisation, and thereafter every subsequent allocation is based on the success or failure of the immediate preceding participant.

173. F Randomisation permutated blocks

This requires randomisation in a group of, say, four, six, etc. to ensure that the numbers are equal in the two groups.

174. D Stratified randomisation

This divides the participants into homogeneous subgroups before sampling. The strata should be mutually exclusive, i.e. every element in the population must be assigned to only one stratum/group. It helps to select representative samples by reducing sampling error. It allocates participants on the basis of the same variables, e.g. prognosis, to ensure that they are evenly distributed within the study. However, it requires an additional schedule for each stratum. Stratification can produce a weighted mean that has less variability compared with the arithmetic mean of a random sample.

175. E Randomised consent method

This is used occasionally to lessen the effect of some patients refusing to participate in a study.

176. C Each participant received both the intervention and the treatment, G Separated by a period of no treatment

Cross-over trials are a real option in relatively rare diseases in which the number of available participants may not permit a randomised, parallel-group, controlled trial. The participants act as their own controls. These trials are useful in psychology, education, pharmaceutical science and medicine (diagnosis, treatment and prevention of disease). They offer two advantages over non-crossover studies: the influence of confounding co-variates is reduced and they are statistically efficient because fewer participants are required. They have several disadvantages: historical controls, 'order', 'learning', and 'carry-over' effects. An n-of-1 trial is a special example of a cross-over trial.

177. B Each group receives a different treatment with both groups being entered at the same time, E Results are analysed by comparing groups

Parallel-group comparison is a part of controlled trials that is necessary to evaluate a new treatment against a placebo or gold standard treatment. This comparison sometimes overestimates the therapeutic benefits.

178. D Participants are assessed before and after an intervention, F Results are analysed in terms of differences between participant pairs

In this type of study design, the participants are offered two alternatives and then asked to indicate to the researchers which alternative they like most. Paired comparison can be included in uncontrolled, controlled and randomised controlled trials of new treatments.

179. A Assumes a poor outcome for drop-outs, E Differences in the drop-out rates and the timing of these drop-outs influence the estimation of treatment

Last observation carried forward (LOCF) is an analytical method used to evaluate a missing value in a clinical trial from the last measurement in an individual participant. Participants who drop out for various reasons, such as side effects or ineffective treatment, are considered treatment failures. LOCF may therefore under- or overestimate the benefits of treatment.

180. D Data on all patients entering a trial should be analysed with respect to the groups to which they were originally randomised. regardless of whether or not they received treatment, E Differences in the drop-out rates and the timing of these drop-outs influence the estimation of treatment

Intention-to-treat analysis is a method to analyse the data generated in the course of a clinical trial according to assigned groups. Trial drop-outs are regarded as treatment failures and cannot be ignored in the analysis of data. All clinical trials should conduct intention-to-treat analysis to avoid overestimating the benefits of treatment. Generally, a continuous measure such as a symptom severity score gives more statistical power than a dichotomous or categorical measure. For a continuous measure, LOCF is used as the final measure.

181. C Data should be analysed as unit of randomisation, F Interventions are directed at groups rather than individual participants

Cluster trials are a special type of RCTs in which interventions are directed at groups rather than individuals. They are commonly used in evaluating more global aspects of health services than one particular treatment, or where allocation of participants is not practicable. They require analysis in clusters, i.e. unit of randomisation rather than individuals, which needs a lot of clusters to detect a statistically significant effect.

182. B Investigations, F Staff salaries

Health economics can be applied to various aspects of healthcare such as treatment. They can help to make decisions about value for money by comparing the effects of competing interventions. An economic analysis requires consideration of the underlying research approach and relevant inputs: direct costs (medical expenses), and indirect costs and inputs. Direct costs are the resources consumed by the programme rather than an alternative.

183. C Pain and suffering, E Social stigma

Intangible costs are immeasurable human costs such as pain, suffering stigma, etc.

184. G Value of 'unpaid work', H Work days lost

Indirect costs are productivity gains and losses with the focus on patient time consumed or freed up by healthcare programmes. They are also referred to as overhead costs, e.g. electricity, gas, rental, capital costs.

185. F Health STAR

Health STAR (Health – Services Technology, Administration and Research) contains materials specifically selected with a focus on health services, research and non-clinical aspects of healthcare delivery (e.g. healthcare administration, economics planning and policy).

186. B CINAHL

The Cumulative Index to Nursing and Allied Health Literature (CINAHL) is a database for nursing literature.

187. D EMBASE

This is a database of pharmaceutical and biomedical literature produced by Elsevier. It concentrates on European sources and drug-related literature. The Cochrane Library is a collection of databases, most of which are solely databases of systematic reviews of healthcare interventions. It provides a quick and focused way of locating RCTs. MEDLINE is a major source of published biomedical scientific literature produced by the National Library of Medicine in the USA. It contains thousands of pieces of published data.

188. D Examples include case reports and series, audits, cross-sectional surveys and qualitative study, F Generally conducted without a control group, H Suitable for hypothesis generation

Descriptive studies are generally conducted without a control group, and are suitable only for generating hypotheses. Examples include case reports, case series, audits, cross-sectional surveys of psychiatric morbidity and qualitative studies.

189. C Examples include case–control and cohort studies, E Generally compare two groups, I Suitable for hypothesis testing

Analytical studies include two groups of participants: cases and controls can be healthy participants or those with a different disease. They are suitable for testing a hypothesis. Examples are case–control studies and cohort studies.

190. A Causation can be inferred, B Examples are controlled clinical trial and economic analyses, systematic reviews and their meta-analyses, G Something is given or done in the experimental group but not in the control group

Experimental studies include 'experimental' and control groups. Any resulting differences in outcome are measured, from which causation may be inferred. Examples of experimental studies are controlled clinical trial and economic analyses, systematic reviews and their meta-analysis.

191. G Single blinding

This helps to reduce potential biases. In a single-blind design, the participants are not aware of the treatment that they are receiving, i.e. placebo or active drug.

192. A Double blinding

In a double-blind study design, both the participants and the investigators are not aware of the treatment that the participants are receiving. This design helps to reduce investigators' bias.

193. G Triple blinding

In this design, the analysis of outcome is carried out by independent investigators who are blind to the treatment given. Both the investigators and the participants are unaware of the treatment that the participants are receiving.

194. D Recall bias

This is introduced by selective memory of participants or informants, who are likely to 'search after meaning' and identify possible exposures. It is also sometimes called 'rumination bias', e.g. depressed patients may be more likely to remember adverse life events. Sometimes, participants may alter their responses in the direction that they perceive is desired by the investigators. This is known as 'obsequiousness bias'.

195. B Incidence risk

This is the number of new cases of a disease over a period of time out of the total population at risk. It is also called cumulative incidence because the number developing disease may change over time through death or loss to follow-up.

196. A Incidence density

This is the new cases of a disease out of the total person-time of observation. It is also called the incidence rate. It provides varying person-years of observation, and is more reliable for quantifying the risk of developing a disease over a certain period of time.

197. E Period prevalence

This includes point prevalence (number of new cases in a population at a particular point in time) and new cases over a period of time.

198. G Standardised mortality ratio

This is calculated as the ratio of observed to expected deaths. It can be analysed by parametric or non-parametric statistics depending on their distribution. The mortality rate is an incidence rate that expresses the risk of death in a population over a period of time. It is useful to have a single measure of mortality for a population to allow meaningful comparison between different populations.

199. D Reduplicative paramnesia

This is the most pathognomonic of brain injury and is also associated with postictal confusional states. The term 'reduplicative paramnesia' covers a range of phenomena, which are often observed concurrently. An example of the phenomenon could be any delusion involving duplication, e.g. that events have been duplicated or that the patient has a second left leg.

200. B Dysprosody

This is a phenomenon in which the normal rhythms and intonations of speech are lost, more so after right hemisphere damage. It interferes with social communication because the voice sounds flat and fails to convey emotion.